Dialysis
Your Passport to Life

by

Dave Capper

Dialysis
Your Passport to Life

by

Dave Capper

ISBN   1492329746

ISBN 13   978-1492329749

Dedication

Over the past several years, I have met many dialysis patients. We became like family, sharing our lives and all of its ups and downs. Smiles and tears. Joy and sorrow. Laughter. Hopes and fears. Good times and bad.

And so I dedicate this book to each of you. You have inspired me to write and to make a difference in people's lives as each of you have made a difference in my life.

Disclaimer

This book is for informational purposes only and nothing in this book is to be considered medical advice. It is recommended and advised that any questions or concerns you have about your health be asked of a medical professional.

Always check with your health care team with any questions or concerns about your health. The general information in this book is not intended to be a substitute for a medical professional.

The use of the name of any product, brand, government agency or company is not an endorsement of that product, brand, government agency or company. All trademarks or names used in this book are the property of its owner and the author makes no representations to the ownership or their respective ownership.

This book is not meant to be used for diagnosis nor treatment of any condition, including, but not limited to, renal failure.

The information in this book, while obtained from reliable sources, should not be relied upon for anything other than basic informational purposes. **Always consult a medical professional about any questions or concerns about your health.**

Table of Contents

Introduction

Renal (kidney) failure affects 20 million Americans with another 20 million at risk. It affects 1 in 5 Canadians, and many more worldwide.

This book will look at what the kidneys do, how they work and what happens when they stop working. We will also look at the many options available once a person's kidneys stop functioning at an effective level.

Prior to 1960, renal failure was not treatable. A person whose kidneys failed would have a short amount of time, less than 30 days, until the fluids and toxins built up in their blood and death would set in.

With the introduction of the dialysis machine, some patients were able to obtain dialysis. The machine was massive and treatment was expensive. During that time, Medicare, Medicaid nor private insurance would not pay for dialysis treatments.

Treatment was not nearly as widely available as it is today. A patient would need to move to wherever a dialysis machine was available, and often times leave family behind, and then only if they were able to pay for the treatments themselves.

With the advancement of technology and treatment payments now offered by private insurance companies, Medicare and Medicaid, patients are able to receive treatment for kidney failure.

While there are different forms of treatment, as of this writing there is no cure for renal failure. With treatments, patients can live a somewhat normal life and live longer.

Some patients are diagnosed at an early age and continue to receive treatments for decades. Older patients, once diagnosed, are able to live longer, healthier lives if they follow a prescribed treatment plan.

I hope this book brings some encouragement to the readers and makes their days a little easier knowing that they are not alone and that options are available.

When things go wrong as they often will, there is a solution for whatever that problem may be. And that when life seems all uphill, remember that a roller coaster ride is also all uphill right before the thrill of the ride.

If you are reading this book, it means you are alive. So I tell you to live every day of your life. Overcome the obstacles in your way and live life to its fullest.

THE KIDNEYS AND HOW THEY WORK

What are the kidneys and what do they do?

The kidneys are two bean-shaped organs, each about the size of a fist. They are located just below the rib cage, one on each side of the spine. Every day, the two kidneys filter about 120 to 150 quarts of blood to produce about 1 to 2 quarts of urine, composed of wastes and extra fluid. The urine flows from the kidneys to the bladder through two thin tubes of muscle called ureters, one on each side of the bladder. The bladder stores urine. The muscles of the bladder wall remain relaxed while the bladder fills with urine. As the bladder fills to capacity, signals sent to the brain tell a person to empty their bladder soon. When the bladder empties, urine flows out of the body through a tube called the urethra, located at the bottom of the bladder. In men, the urethra is long while in women it is short.

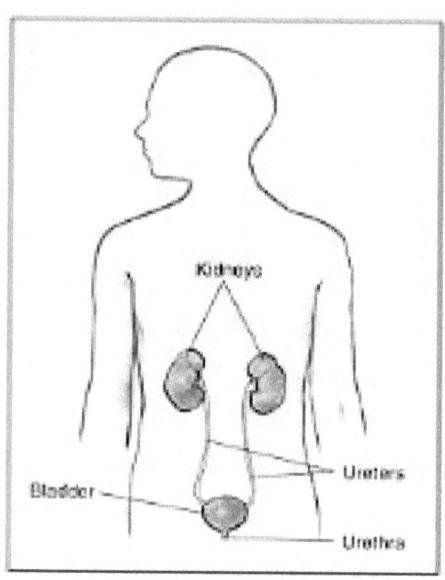

The urinary tract

Why are the kidneys important?

The kidneys are important because they keep the composition, or makeup, of the blood stable, which lets the body function. They

- prevent the buildup of wastes and extra fluid in the body
- keep levels of electrolytes stable, such as sodium, potassium, and phosphate
make hormones that regulate

    - blood pressure
    - red blood cells
    - bone turnover, which may increase the risk for bone fractures.

- An imbalance may affect your bone, heart, and blood vessels.

How do the kidneys work?

The kidney is not one large filter. In fact, each kidney is made up of about a million filtering units called nephrons. Each nephron filters a small amount of blood. The nephron includes a filter, called the glomerulus, and a tubule. The nephrons work through a two-step process. The glomerulus lets fluid and waste products pass through it; however, it prevents blood cells and large molecules, mostly proteins, from passing. The filtered fluid then passes through the tubule, which reabsorbs what as needed, and removes the rest as urine.

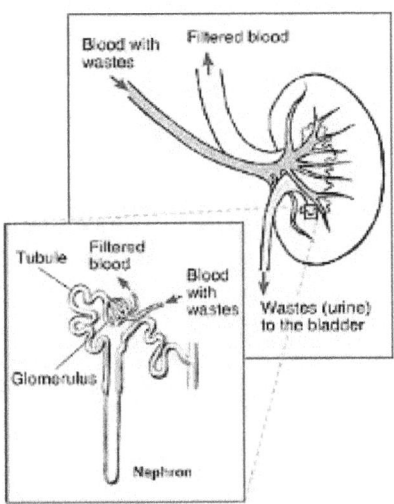

Each kidney is made up of about a million filtering units called nephrons.

Points to Remember

- Every day, the two kidneys filter about 120 to 150 quarts of blood to produce about 1 to 2 quarts of urine, composed of wastes and extra fluid.
- The kidneys are important because they keep the composition, or makeup, of the blood stable, which lets the body function.

- Each kidney is made up of about a million filtering units called nephrons. The nephron includes a filter, called the glomerulus, and a tubule.
- The nephrons work through a two-step process. The glomerulus lets fluid and waste products pass through it; however, it prevents blood cells and large molecules, mostly proteins, from passing. The filtered fluid then passes through the tubule, which sends needed minerals back to the bloodstream and removes wastes.

The information above is provided by The National Kidney and Urologic Diseases Information Clearinghouse (NKUDIC).

TYPES OF TREATMENT

Dialysis

Dialysis is the only form of treatment other than to do nothing for kidney failure. When the kidneys stop working or work less than they once did, a decision will need to be made to visit a nephrologist, (kidney doctor). The nephrologist will determine the best course of action in your case. Each case is different though perhaps in many ways treatments for different patients may seem the same. A treatment plan will be made specifically for you as you work with the nephrologist to determine what is right for you. Periodically, your treatment plan will be reviewed and adjusted as needed by the dialysis staff and your nephrologist.

Treatment can be either temporary or permanent dialysis to a kidney transplant. Dialysis offers many different options to choose from. You and your nephrologist can determine which is best for you.

This book is about the dialysis treatment and the dialysis access needed for dialysis. Kidney transplants are not discussed in great detail in this book, although dialysis may be used until you receive a transplant if your treatment plan includes a possible transplant.

Once you have met with your nephrologist, they will discuss with you the different options available that best suits you. Whatever your treatment plan is, remember to always take it seriously and follow through on all aspects of the treatment plan.

Dialysis in a Clinic

Your treatment options will most likely include dialysis, temporary or permanent, and you will be given a few different options for that treatment. One of those options will be in-clinic dialysis. The in-clinic dialysis is an option for virtually all renal failure patients, although not the only option for dialysis for most. There are treatment centers throughout the United States and the world. Many hospitals offer dialysis for acute renal failure hospitalized kidney patients, end stage renal disease patients and emergencies. Those needing emergency dialysis, such as the case of trauma for instance, may also find treatment available at a local hospital. Some hospitals may be the only dialysis center in the area, and all of your treatments may be at the hospital. Some areas have several in-clinic sites available and different providers. Once a treatment plan is decided, you and your nephrologist can then decide on which treatment location may be best for you.

Dialysis can be permanent or temporary. Most are permanent and if so, you may need to take dialysis treatments three days a week for the rest of your life. Others are temporary. Temporary can mean the kidneys are functioning well enough after a series of treatments, or you may have received a kidney transplant. Whether you are to receive permanent or temporary dialysis will be determined by your nephrologist and will be evaluated again after you have had several treatments and again periodically as treatment plans are re-evaluated by the dialysis team and nephrologist.

If the decision is made to have dialysis in a treatment center, whether temporary or permanent, you will need to make arrangements for transportation to each treatment. Some areas may offer free or reduced rates when using a local transportation system. Some clinics have a driver and vehicle that will pick you up for each treatment and return you home afterward. Ultimately, it is your responsibility to get to treatments. It is never advisable to miss any treatments or to leave treatments early. This can affect the quality of your treatments and will cause complications and even shorten your life expectancy. This is discussed in more detail later in this chapter.

Most dialysis patients need three treatments each week. These are done on Monday, Wednesday, and Friday or Tuesday, Thursday and Saturday. In-center dialysis is best if done every other day allowing the body to recover and still not have a long period between treatments allowing toxins and fluids to build up to dangerous levels.

You will need to determine which schedule is best for you and advise the nephrologist prior to being assigned to a clinic. Changing from one schedule to another can be difficult, as dialysis centers are busy and need to make room for you on any given shift or day. A shift, for dialysis sake, is 4 hours. When someone refers to first shift, for example, they may mean appointment times from 6 am until 10 am time slots. Many dialysis centers schedule patients every 15 minutes to allow time to connect and disconnect patients to or from a dialysis machine before the next patient's appointment time. In doing this, you may or may not be placed on a machine the exact time each day. The staff can fall behind as the day progresses for a variety of reasons. Bring a book or something to do while on dialysis. It can be a long 4 hours if there is nothing to do.

What will happen now?

Once a location is established for your treatment, here are a few things you should know:

- Most patients will have three treatments a week.

- Each treatment will be from 3 or more hours.

- Your dialysis center will give you an appointment time that will be your time.

- Wear the same clothing to each treatment. Clothes can become damaged by blood or the bleach or other chemicals used by the staff to clean chairs and equipment. Wearing the same clothes with each treatment can also mean more accurate weigh in and weigh out weights.

It is imperative that you not miss or skip any dialysis appointments. Missing an appointment will cause complications for you. Your kidneys have stopped functioning and treatments are the only way for fluids and waste to be removed, a job that was once done by the kidneys. Missing or shortening treatments will cause your body to fill with fluids and waste which are harmful. Dialysis works best only if you are being dialyzed completely with each treatment and not miss, shorten or postpone treatments.

Dialysis will account only about 10 to 15 percent of the work your kidneys once did. Your kidneys worked 24 hours a day using millions of nephrons, or filters, and dialysis is the use of a machine during a 4 hour period three days a week. Missing treatments will cause complications and will shorten your life considerably with each missed appointment. Always keep your appointments and allow the machines the time they need to keep you healthier.

You will be asked to make up any missed or shortened treatments the next day. It can also cause all other patients scheduled after you to be delayed. So take care of yourself and remember to be respectful of others and keep the appointments and arrive on time. If, for some reason, you are unable to make a scheduled appointment, call the clinic and advise them giving them as much notice as you can allowing them to reschedule other patients.

Dialysis is a process allowing a machine to filter and remove waste and excess fluids. This process takes about 4 hours, and it needs to be repeated three times a week, or in some cases, more often.

Prior to your appointment time, you may have been prescribed a numbing agent. Many patients use this numbing agent over the access area to prevent pain or discomfort when inserting the needles for their dialysis treatment. Ask your nephrologist about this prior to the first treatment. Inserting the needles can be uncomfortable and the numbing agent can ease that discomfort. If you are using the numbing agent, apply the cream and then loosely wrap the area in a plastic wrap. Do not wrap the arm tightly. Remember, if a numbing agent is used, it must be applied at least 45 minutes prior to treatment to allow it to absorb and be most effective.

You may be given an appointment with a dialysis center if this is the location where your dialysis is to take place. Once you are at the dialysis center, the staff will do the following:

- They will weigh you before and after each treatment. The initial weight will allow the staff to know an approximate amount of excess fluids you may have had prior to treatment. Your current weight minus your dry weight, once it is determined, will determine how much excess fluid you may have that the dialysis machine needs to remove, along with the wastes.

- The access area needs to be cleaned prior to treatment. Washing the access area it is also advisable even when you choose not to use a numbing agent as described above.

- They will check your vital signs, including blood pressure, temperature and heart rate.

- Needles will be placed in your access area to allow blood to flow in and out. The needles may be uncomfortable at first. You can ask the provider for a numbing cream prescription if you are not currently using one, (as discussed above) if the needles are uncomfortable.

- Once your treatment is over, the staff will remove the needles, ask you to put pressure on the site and after a period of time, place a dressing on your access area and weigh you once again.

The needles and tubing that connects to the dialysis machine will transport your blood into the dialysis machine, where the blood is filtered, excess fluids and wastes removed, and blood placed back into your body.

Your dialysis treatments will usually last from 3 or hours, but this will be determined by your treatment plan. Some patients may need less time for each dialysis treatment while others need more time for treatment. You may need a longer treatment if you have excess fluids on a particular day.

During treatment, you will need something to occupy your time. Talking to other patients or reading a book perhaps will pass the time quicker.

You will probably feel tired after your treatments and will need a recovery period. While some people need an hour or so to rest, someone else may need more or less time. And you may need more time after one treatment than you may need after another treatment. Do not overdo things and take whatever time you need to recover. You can go home and rest for the rest of the day if need be. Your body will tell you how much rest you will need. Let your body guide you on how much rest you need. Do not schedule anything other than dialysis on treatment day.

After your first several treatments, you may experience some nausea, cramping, dizziness, and or headaches. The symptoms will likely go away after a few treatments. Always tell your dialysis staff of any discomfort you may be experiencing either while on the dialysis machine or at other times. They may be able to adjust your treatment plan or provide some relief for whatever the discomfort may be.

Too much fluid in your body can cause certain symptoms such as difficulty breathing, swelling of the ankles or legs, or sleepiness. Consult with your dialysis staff or doctors if you are experiencing any of these symptoms.

The length of the treatment you will need each time is determined by some factors:

- How well your kidneys are functioning;

- Your weight when you check in for treatment will be a factor. Ideally the goal is to bring you down to your dry weight, or slightly below your dry weight after your treatment;

- How much waste needs to be removed? Once again, this is determined by dry weight as well.

- Whether or not you still have residual kidney function, while those who do not have residual kidney function will retain more fluid which needs to be removed with the dialysis machine during a treatment.

Between sessions

Dialysis is only a part of your treatment plan. There may need to be some changes to your daily routine. A person whose kidneys have failed may find they do not urinate as often as they once did. Some dialysis patients may no longer urinate at all. If fluids are not being removed through urination, excess fluids will build up in the body faster than those who urinate with normal frequency and or in normal amounts. Some patients experience little change in urination frequency. The urination frequency can change over time. Let the dialysis staff know of any changes in urination frequency, as this can affect your treatment, fluid restriction levels and diet.

Excess fluids can lead to congestive heart failure, among other complications. Fluid can build up around the heart, and the heart then has little or no room to move as it does when it pumps blood normally. The heart then has to work harder in a confined space and eventually it cannot pump blood. Once this happens, the heart can slow to a dangerous pace or stop altogether. When fluids build up around the heart, causing the heart not to pump normally, it is called cardiac tamponade. Cardiac tamponade is a serious condition when the blood or fluid builds up in a space between the sac that encases the heart and the heart muscle. This restriction can cause the heart to work harder or even stop.

Other complications can occur when a person has excess fluid as well. You may be more tired than usual. Being tired is normal, but you need to talk to the dialysis staff about this.

With advances in dialysis today, as opposed to years ago, you are no longer restricted to one clinic for treatment. You are free to travel and can receive dialysis at many different dialysis centers around the world. Of course, traveling will depend on whether you are up to traveling. You will need to set this up in advance to make appointments along your journey for dialysis treatments. Some home clinics may make all of the necessary arrangements if you give them a copy of your travel plans. Insurance plans may pay the same as they would at your home clinic. Do not assume insurance will pay at different locations, and so you are advised to check with your insurance carrier to determine if they will pay or if you will be required to pay for any treatments while traveling.

Believe it or not, you can even take a cruise. That's right. Dialysis cruises are available. You will need to book the cruise and while onboard, have a dialysis treatment in the onboard clinic with dialysis staff onboard the ship. You will need to inquire about the costs and whether or not your insurance will pay for the dialysis portion of the cruise. Your dialysis staff may be able to help you with making these arrangements as well. (Isn't the dialysis staff amazing)?

When to call your doctor

With dialysis, you will find your body is adjusting to the changes. With each treatment, you should begin to feel better and while this is a good thing, do not mistake feeling better with being cured. You feel better because of the treatments, and it is not a cure for kidney disease. Therefore, remember to keep each dialysis appointment and stay for the entire treatment. It would only take a few missed treatments over a short period to feel poor again. Missing treatments or signing out early will shorten your life span. You will need each full treatment to remove the fluids and waste that have built up in your body since your last treatment. Again, never mistake feeling better as a sign you do not need to have treatment. The longer fluids and waste build up in your body, the more damage it will do to the organs and it will shorten your life span.

There is also a time when you may not feel well or just not feel like yourself. If this happens, you will need to know when to call the doctor or the dialysis clinic. You will re-learn your body over time and know what is normal and what is not normal. Until then, call the dialysis clinic and they can advise you more on whatever your concern is. Communicate with them and they can help you through the adjustments. If they do not know, they cannot help you.

The times when you need to call will be if you notice any of the following:

- Any bleeding from your access site. Excessive bleeding requires applying pressure to stop the bleeding and immediately calling 911.

- Any signs of infection, such as redness, swelling, soreness, pain, warmth, or pus around the site

- A fever over 100°

- The location of your catheter becomes swollen, tender or warm

- Your hand gets cold, numb, or weak

You will need to call your doctor or dialysis center if you suffer from any of the following symptoms for more than a day or two:

- Diarrhea ,

- Nauseated or vomiting,

- Confusion, (unable to concentrate) more so than before beginning dialysis.

"When in doubt, give a shout" is a good rule to remember.

Home Dialysis

There are two forms of home dialysis. The first, which we will discuss in this section, is similar to the treatment offered during an in-clinic setting. The other is peritoneal dialysis, which is discussed later in this chapter. For purposes of clarity, this book refers to home dialysis as that treatment which is administered by the patient, or caregiver, at home with the use of a dialysis machine. The term "Peritoneal" will be used when referring to a dialysis treatment through the abdomen and into the peritoneal cavity of the body. Both can be completed at home and are considered home dialysis.

You will have a home dialysis training team. This team will be made up of professionals who will train and assist you. They will answer any questions you may have. The team consists of your kidney doctor (nephrologist), a training nurse, a social worker, a renal dietitian, patient care technicians, and machine and water technicians.

Your training team has been trained to help train you and guide you throughout the process. Each will play a vital role in making home dialysis as trouble free as possible.

Some things you will need:

1. A clean room or area in your home,

2. Space for dialysis supplies and equipment,

3. Storage space for 6 weeks of supplies.

4. A bed or chair in which you will be during your treatment, and

5. Good lighting

You will receive all of the equipment and supplies you will need for 4 to 6 weeks of treatment. The exact things you will receive will depend on the type of treatment and location of your treatment. Your home dialysis training nurse will go over this with you. Some of the items will include:

1. Dialysis machine,

2. Sharps container for disposal of needles and other hazardous material,

3. Tubing as needed for dialysis,

4. Dialysis solution (dialysate).

You will need to keep a set of records. The records will include treatment records, machine and water testing log, medications, and a list of any calls you have made to someone about the dialysis concerns you may have. The purpose of the list of concerns is so that when you visit the clinic monthly, they can review those concerns with you in more detail if needed.

You will visit the home dialysis clinic once a month. At that time, they will go over lab reports, changes that need to be made or questions that you may have. They will review your records and discuss them with you during this visit as well.

Bring your records and the sharps container, if more than ¾ full, with you. They will dispose of the container for you. If you are in need of a new container, they can provide one for you.

You will need to know how much or how little supplies you have on hand. It will be your responsibility to order new supplies when needed. Your training nurse can tell you how to order new supplies when needed. Remember to allow time for shipping and delivery.

Nocturnal Dialysis

Nocturnal dialysis is dialysis at night while you sleep. It can be an option for those who have an active life or perhaps have no transportation available during the day. For instance, some patients have a job and continue to work after being placed on dialysis. If you work a job or have other things to do during the day, or maybe transportation is a problem during the day, you may be a candidate for nocturnal dialysis.

Nocturnal dialysis can be done at home or in-clinic. Some clinics offer nocturnal dialysis. If your clinic does not offer nocturnal dialysis, and you are interested in learning more about this type of dialysis, ask your nephrologist or dialysis staff for information about whether or not this type of treatment is offered in your area. Not all clinics offer nocturnal dialysis, but it may be available in your area at a different location.

The nocturnal treatment is virtually the same as in-clinic dialysis (discussed above) although it is performed overnight while you sleep, allowing you to continue with daytime activities.

One difference is that the length of the treatments may be longer than that of in clinic dialysis. This form of dialysis can take 7 to 8 hours, while in-clinic dialysis may be approximately half of that time. By removing fluids and wastes over a longer period of time, it can be less of a strain on other organs, including the heart.

Nocturnal dialysis can be done in your home however, will need a care partner available during treatments to assist you or to be available in the case of complications. Because of needing a care partner, nocturnal home dialysis may not be an option.

Peritoneal Dialysis

There are two types of peritoneal dialysis, Continuous Ambulatory Peritoneal Dialysis, (CAPD) and Continuous Cycling Peritoneal Dialysis (CCPD).

CAPD does not require a machine. It is referred to as a manual form of dialysis. A double bag system is used. One bag contains dialysate which is placed above the head, allowing gravity to feed the fluids into the peritoneal cavity. Some CAPD patients use an intravenous pole to hang the bag of dialysate similar to what you would see in a hospital.

The second bag is empty and is placed on the floor to catch the fluids as they are removed from the body by opening a valve or unclamping the tubing leading to the bag. Once the first bag is empty, it can be turned off or clamped. The dialysate will remain in the peritoneal cavity for about 4 hours. It is then drained into the second bag by opening the valve or clamp to the second bag. Once the second bag is full, the flow can be turned off by using the clamp or valve on the tubing.

This is called an exchange. Once the exchange is complete, you carefully disconnect from the tubing.

You then empty the full bag into a toilet to dispose of the contents by opening the valve or clamp and draining the contents into a toilet. Once this is done, clamp the tubing and discard the bags and tubing in your trash. This process is repeated every 4 to 5 hours each day.

Needles and syringes must be placed in a sharps container which is provided by your dialysis equipment supplier and disposed of by taking them to the home dialysis clinic during your monthly visit.

There are pros and cons of this type of treatment.

The pros are:

1. No need for a machine,

2. Can be done virtually anywhere,

The cons are:

1. It must be done each day.

2. An exchange may take approximately 1 hour,

3. And the CAPD must be repeated every 4 to 5 hours during the day.

While CAPD is manual and does not use any machine, CCPD uses a machine, called a cycler, to perform dialysis. These cycles are done during the night while you sleep. While you sleep, the machine will automatically fill and drain the dialysate from the peritoneal cavity.

As with CAPD, disposing of the drained bags, gauze, gloves, medication bottles and masks used for CCPD can also be disposed of with your regular trash. Needles and syringes must be placed in a sharps container which is provided by your dialysis equipment supplier and disposed of by taking them to the home dialysis clinic during your monthly visit. Disposing of fluids is as easy as draining into the toilet, as described above with the use of CAPD.

With either type, peritoneal dialysis is a process involving a dialysis solution (dialysate) being placed in the abdominal cavity (the peritoneal cavity) within the lining of the belly using a permanent catheter. The dialysate will remain in the cavity for a period of time, allowing it to trap the wastes. After a period of time, the dialysate is then removed from the lower abdomen along with the waste and disposed. This process can take place anywhere a person has a clean area in their home or office, or virtually anywhere. It does require a relatively large, dry, area to store supplies for this type of treatment.

Peritoneal dialysis allows a patient to do their dialysis virtually anywhere and on their schedule. Not all patients can do peritoneal dialysis. Ask your nephrologists if this is an option for you.

CAPD and CCPD similarities:

1. Both CAPD and CCPD use peritoneal catheters for access,

2. Both are done at home, or virtually anywhere the patient may be.

CAPD and CCPD differences:

1. CAPD must be repeated several times each day while CCPD is done during sleep,

2. CAPD is manually performed while CCPD is done with the use of a machine.

DIALYSIS ACCESS TYPES

Over the last few decades, life expectancy has been significantly improved with the advent of dialysis access types such as arteriovenous fistula ("fistula"), central venous catheters ("catheters"), and arteriovenous grafts ("grafts"). In this chapter, we will look at these three main types of dialysis accesses.

There are three main types of access which can provide access for your dialysis. The type of access you will have will depend on your needs and will be determined by your doctor. They will determine which access is best suited in your case by using multiple test results.

This chapter will discuss each of those types and how each access device works. There are, of course, pros and cons of each type and that, too, will be discussed. People tend to feel afraid or anxious about the unknown. Your nephrologist will know what is best for you and will direct your care with that in mind.

The first of the three access types is the catheter, or Central Venous Catheter (CVC) which is a temporary access used primarily while the permanent access matures, which will then be ready for treatments.

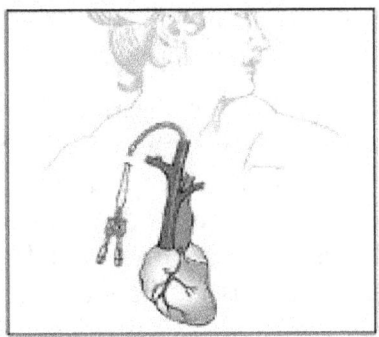

Central Venous Catheter

For Hemodialysis, the catheter is generally placed in the arm or neck. However, there are times when it will need to be in other areas, such as the groin.

Ultrasound Guided Catheter Placement

One of the more common ways to place a catheter is with the use of the Utlrasound guided catheter placement procedure. This procedure allows the surgeon to view the catheter during insertion avoiding complications. In some instances, such as an emergency procedure, or in the case where ultrasound equipment is not available, a practitioner may insert the catheter with what is sometimes referred to as a blind catheter placement.

Ultrasound guided catheter placement is a procedure that allows the practitioner to view the veins as they insert the catheter allowing them to track the path of the catheter during insertion.

Central Venous Catheter (CVC)

Your first access will likely be a central venous catheter. For this, you will need an ultrasound of the area that will assist the surgeon in determining the best location for the placement of the catheter. The ultrasound is the same as described above for vein mapping.

The catheter can be inserted into the chest or the leg, depending on your body's ability to accept a catheter. Most catheters are placed into the chest although the catheter can be inserted in the neck or groin as determined by the surgeon. The catheter can be used almost immediately after placement. The purpose of the catheter is to allow a temporary access until the permanent type of access has matured and can be used. Catheter accesses allow dialysis through the catheter and are not to be used permanently as this causes a higher rate of infection and other complications that can occur from extended use of a catheter.

The surgeon will insert the catheter through a small incision in your skin. The catheter is placed into a vein. When completed, the surgeon will use stitches to hold the catheter in place until it heals. Once it is healed, generally two weeks after placement, the stitches can be removed.

It is a relatively simple procedure that should only take a short time, usually slightly more than an hour. The placing of a catheter will need to be done in a hospital, surgical center, or procedure center. Once the catheter procedure has been completed, you may have a dialysis treatment almost immediately, unlike other accesses that require more healing time to allow use. Once your permanent access is placed and used, it may clot or have other complications. If this happens, a new catheter may be used until a new permanent access can mature.

You may have a permanent type of access created or implanted the same day of the catheter placement. However, your surgeon will tell you how long you will need to use the catheter before attempting to use the other type of access.

Once the catheter is in place, you may then receive your dialysis treatments using the catheter until the dialysis clinic staff, following the advice of the surgeon, or your nephrologist tells you otherwise. The staff will use the new access site, a fistula or graft, a number of times prior to making an appointment for you to have the catheter removed. Using the permanent access allows them to be certain the access will work properly without any complications prior to removing your catheter. Long-term use of a catheter can cause complications, such as infection.

Removing the catheter will not be done at the dialysis clinic but rather generally, the same, or similar, facility where the catheter placement procedure took place. That location will be either in a hospital, surgical center or a procedure center. The procedure takes a shorter time than the time to insert a catheter, and you will be able to go home once the catheter has been removed.

A new catheter can be inserted again at a later time should it become necessary, for instance in a case where a permanent access becomes unusable for some reason. Again, this will be temporary access until the permanent access becomes available to use.

Vein Mapping

Vein mapping is the use of ultrasound or angiography to find the veins that will be available for dialysis access. A map of your veins and arteries need to be completed prior to placing your access to assure it is placed correctly and in the best place for your successful treatments. Not all veins can be used for dialysis access and with the use of vein mapping the surgeon can determine which veins are best for you.

Vein mapping is done using ultrasound. It is painless, not invasive and simply requires a mapping of the veins with the use of a machine to find the best veins when searching for the best access site. It does not require any surgery. The vein mapping may be done right in your doctor's office in a matter of minutes without any pain or discomfort at all.

An ultrasound is simply a machine allowing for a view of the veins using a gel on the skin and a wand type mechanism. The technician will place some gel on the area to be mapped. They will then glide the wand over the skin giving a reading of the veins on a monitor. You will hear the sounds of blood flowing through the veins from the monitor, and the technician will make a recording of the veins. It is painless and takes only a few minutes to complete.

Unlike the ultrasound, an angiography or angiogram is invasive. An angiography or angiogram is done by inserting a catheter into the vein allowing the surgeon to insert a dye. The surgeon then can view the veins using x-ray. The X-ray allows the surgeon to locate the best veins to use for dialysis access.

Once the veins have been located, and it is determined which veins give the best chance of success, a fistula is created.

Arteriovenous Fistula (AVF)

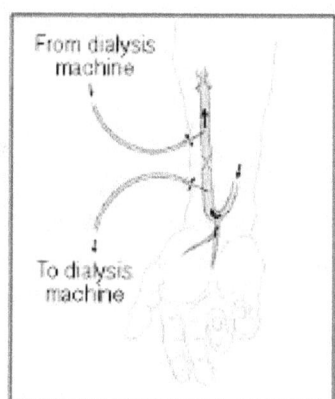

To create a fistula, the doctors will need to know which vein is best for your success. Determining where to insert the access will be done with the use of vein mapping.

Another common type of dialysis access is an arteriovenous fistula. The arteriovenous fistula is more commonly referred to simply as a fistula. A fistula is the most common type of access for most dialysis patients. In the case of dialysis, it is a connection between an artery and a vein making access for dialysis possible. With dialysis, there need to be vessels large enough to handle the blood flow in and out. Normal sized vessels are not always large enough to handle that much flow, and so a fistula may be needed.

An AV fistula is a connection, made by a surgeon, of an artery to a vein. Arteries carry blood from the heart to the body, while veins carry blood from the body back to the heart. Vascular surgeons specialize in blood vessel surgery. The surgeon usually places an AV fistula in the forearm or upper arm. An AV fistula causes extra pressure and extra blood to flow into the vein, making it grow large and strong. The larger vein provides easy, reliable access to blood vessels. Without this kind of access, regular hemodialysis sessions would not be possible. Untreated veins cannot withstand repeated needle insertions. They would collapse the way a straw collapses under strong suction.

Health care providers recommend an AV fistula over the other types of access because it:

- provides good blood flow for dialysis

- lasts longer than other types of access

- is less likely to get infected or cause blood clots than other types of access

Before AV fistula surgery, the surgeon may perform a vessel mapping test. Vessel mapping uses Doppler ultrasound to evaluate blood vessels that the surgeon may use to make the

AV fistula. Ultrasound uses a device, called a transducer that bounces safe, painless sound waves off organs to create an image of their structure. A specially trained technician performs the procedure in a health care provider's office, an outpatient center, or a hospital. A radiologist—a doctor who specializes in medical imaging—interprets the images. A patient does not need anesthesia. A Doppler ultrasound shows how much and how quickly blood flows through arteries and veins so the surgeon can select the best blood vessels to use.

A surgeon performs AV fistula surgery in an outpatient center or a hospital. The vascular access procedure may require an overnight stay in the hospital; however, many patients go home afterward. A health care provider uses local anesthesia to numb the area where the surgeon creates the AV fistula.

An AV fistula frequently requires 2 to 3 months to develop, or mature, before the patient can use it for hemodialysis. If an AV fistula fails to mature after surgery, a surgeon must repeat the procedure.

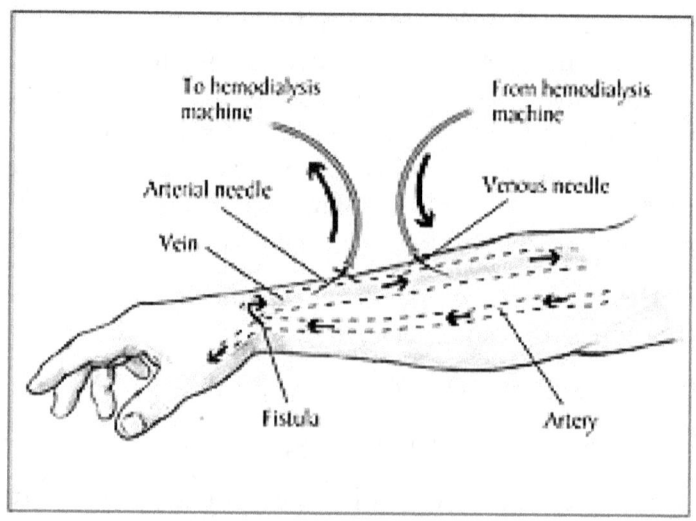

To hemodialysis machine

From hemodialysis machine

Arterial needle

Venous needle

Vein

Fistula

Artery

AV fistula in forearm

At the start of a hemodialysis session, a health care provider or the patient inserts two needles into the vascular access. One needle carries blood from the body to the dialyzer.

The other carries filtered blood back to the body. To tell the needles apart, the needle that carries blood away from the body is called the arterial needle. The needle that carries blood back to the body is called the venous needle. Some patients prefer to insert their own needles into the vascular access, which requires training to learn how to prevent infection and protect the vascular access. No matter who inserts the needles, the patient should know how to take care of the needle insertion area to prevent infection.

If an AV fistula does not mature, or your veins cannot be used for access for any reason, an AV graft is the second choice for a long-lasting vascular access.

Buttonhole Cannulation

The use of the buttonhole cannulation is when the dialysis team uses the same two holes at each treatment, much like those found on the button on a shirt.

Constant-Site Access

See Buttonhole Cannulation section above

Rope-Ladder Technique

The rope ladder technique is the preferred method of needling (using needles in the graft or fistula with each treatment). Simply put, it means to use a different location on the graft or fistula with each treatment so as not to wear out the access, allowing it time to seal before using that location again. As opposed to the buttonhole cannulation discussed above, where it is required to use the same hole at precisely the same angle with each treatment, the rope-ladder technique requires the use of different locations along the access to avoid wearing the access out or puncturing the access. It is likely called the rope-ladder technique because of the pattern used for access.

The rope ladder is most often the preferred type of access in a clinic. A self-needling person, one who may choose to do home dialysis, for example, may prefer the buttonhole cannulation. Ask your nephrologist if this is an option for you.

Arteriovenous Graft

An AV graft, or "graft," is a looped, plastic tube that connects an artery to a vein. A vascular surgeon performs AV graft surgery, much like AV fistula surgery, in an outpatient center or a hospital. As with AV fistula surgery, AV Graft surgery may require the patient to stay overnight in the hospital. Many patients can go home after the procedure. A health care provider uses local anesthesia to numb the area where the surgeon creates the AV graft.

A patient can usually use an AV graft two to three weeks after the surgery. An AV graft is more likely than an AV fistula to have problems with infection and clotting. Repeated blood clots can block the flow of blood through the graft. However, a well-cared-for graft can last several years.

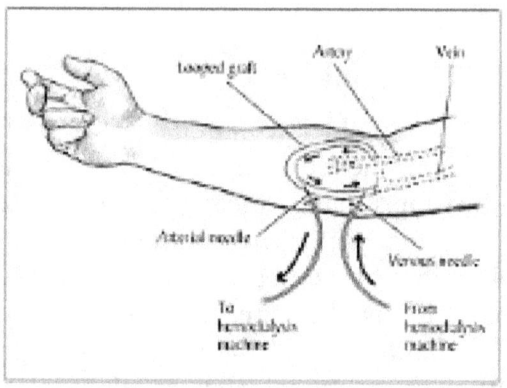

AV graft in forearm

Peritoneal

Before your first treatment, a surgeon places a catheter into your abdomen (peritoneal cavity). The catheter tends to work better if there is adequate time-usually from 10 days to 2 or 3 weeks-for the insertion site to heal. Planning your dialysis access can improve treatment success. This catheter stays there permanently to help transport the dialysis solution to and from your abdomen.

Pros and Cons

Each patient is different. Not every patient can use all of the various forms of access and, therefore over time, different means of access have been developed for dialysis. It has been said that necessity is the mother of invention. As patients needed a different type of dialysis, someone invented a new way to accommodate them. You may also find your form of access or treatment changing over time. Doctors and the dialysis staff will make decisions as needed to provide you the best possible treatment to suit your needs.

With each form of access, there are pros and cons. Your medical team can discuss in more detail the different types and which may be best for you in your particular situation. Never assume that one is better than another as it depends on your veins and how well you tolerate dialysis and a number of variables. For instance if you have good veins, you may be a candidate for buttonhole cannulation access while someone else may fare better with the use of a graft or a fistula. You can discuss these different types with your medical team, and they can determine which is best for you. You and your medical team will need to choose the best option for you based on your individual needs.

Dialysis is not a one size fits all nor are the different types of accesses a one size fits all solution. But there is an access type for you and a dialysis type that will work best for you. The different types of access allow options when other accesses may not available to them.

The number and types of access allow more flexibility for a patient. The use of one over another being better or worse depends on the patient and their body. The best possible access could be your veins whether using a buttonhole cannulation or a fistula.

It is always the best policy to trust those who treat you to do so with your best interest in mind and for you to follow the treatment plan as set for you. Your medical team is well trained and has experience in all aspects of kidney failure and dialysis. You will need to trust them to make good choices and follow their guidance.

Remember that it is important to stay for the entire prescribed treatment and do not miss treatments. Studies have shown that patients who miss treatments or sign out early from treatments are at higher risk for complications and even death. No one wants to be on dialysis, but people who require dialysis need this treatment to survive and to stay healthier. Missing or shortening treatments will lead to more medical problems for the patient and eventually can lead to death if a person is missing their dialysis appointments or signing out early from treatments. You are going to be scheduled for a certain amount of time for each treatment to allow the dialysis machine to remove toxins and fluids. If you choose to leave early or miss treatments, all of the toxins and fluids are not removed and remain in your body. Missing treatments or signing out early and not completing treatments allows more toxins and fluid to build up in your body and this is not healthy. The purpose of dialysis is to remove the toxins and fluid and leaving early and not allowing the time needed will lessen the treatment success.

Treatments in a center can lead to new friendships. For a patient, for instance, who cannot get out of the house often, this can be a refreshing time. You will learn from each other and form a bond with others that few will understand.

In a smaller community, you may find several people you already know and in larger communities you will form new friendships with others who have similar experiences with their health. Be friends with them and learn to work together through your common issues. When a person is sick, we believe no one understands what we are experiencing. With dialysis, the patients know what you are going through and can help you through it.

It can never be said enough to always to keep your dialysis appointments and NEVER sign out early.

PROTECTING YOUR ACCESS

Vascular access is the means of administering your dialysis. It is extremely important to protect it from being damaged. In this section, we will look at some of the ways you will need to protect it and how you can check it yourself at home, or wherever you may be.

Once you are told you will need dialysis, your first means of access will likely be a catheter through which the dialysis staff can access the bloodstream to perform the dialysis treatments. A catheter is placed in the chest area but may also be placed in the leg or another area. It is a tube placed in the chest, or other places that can be used depending on your body and arteries. The location of your catheter and other permanent access will be decided by your surgeon after vein mapping and other considerations. The catheter has a single tube on one end and connected to a double access tube that is used to insert needles for dialysis. One tube will be red and the other blue.

One tube will be used for drawing blood out of the body and into the dialysis machine, and the other for returning the blood to the body once the dialysis machine has removed fluids and toxins from the blood. The blood is chilled during this process so you may feel cold during dialysis and for a while after dialysis until your body has warmed the blood once again. Being cold during dialysis is not unusual. You may wish to bring a light blanket to dialysis or wear warm clothes to each treatment, but remember only to wear short sleeves to allow the staff to use your access easily.

The catheter should remain covered with gauze and tape when not in use at dialysis. However, during treatments, it should remain visible to the staff to allow them to monitor the catheter. The catheter needs to remain clean. It is very important that you keep the catheter clean and sterile. The catheter is inserted into the main bloodstream, an artery, and any infection can be serious, and even fatal.

The catheter should not get wet. It is advisable not to shower after the catheter is placed. Moisture or dampness can allow bacteria to grow, and this can cause infection in and around the catheter. This infection can get into the blood stream that can cause sepsis. Sepsis is an infection of the blood. Sepsis, left untreated, can be fatal.

You may also have a fistula or graft placed the same day. The graft or fistula will need time to mature before being used for dialysis treatments. During this time, the dialysis staff will use the catheter.

Once your access is placed, you will need to follow a few very simple rules.

- Always keep it covered with gauze and tape.

- Do not shower or get the access site wet until it has healed completely and you are told by your dialysis team otherwise.

- Do not disturb any scabbing around the site. Let it heal on its own and any scabbing will naturally come off of the skin.

- Call your dialysis center if area around the catheter site becomes red or swollen.

- If you notice any light bleeding or pus around the access site, call the dialysis center or in the case of heavy or uncontrolled bleeding, call 911 immediately.

You will also need to pay careful attention to others who are around you and your access so that they do not unintentionally cause damage to your access.

Some things you did prior to having an access may need to be limited or eliminated completely. Your dialysis staff can advise you on limiting or eliminating activities.

Putting too much pressure on the access can cause it to become damaged and or slow down, or even stop the blood flow through the access causing you to need intervention or even a new access.

Wear loose clothing over the access area. Wearing tight clothes over the access can put pressure on the access and can cause the access not to work requiring intervention or a new access being needed.

You may use clothing specifically made for dialysis, or have a seamstress make special clothing for you. The clothing may be a shirt or a blouse you have used prior to dialysis, with the sleeves cut along the seam. Instead of sewing them back together, use Velcro or snaps to allow the dialysis staff to open them easily to access the dialysis access site. Once dialysis is completed, the shirt or blouse simply Velcro or snap back together. By wearing these clothes, you are easily able to access the site and once treatment is completed, you can cover the arm keeping it warm.

Be cautious when using the access arm for any activities. Always be mindful of where the access is.

Do not bother scabs that may be forming over the access area. Scabbing is the normal process of healing. Scabbing allows the body to grow new skin tissues and will protect the wound from infection. If you disturb the scabs, it can cause bleeding, and this can become uncontrollable bleeding. Leave them alone and let the site heal. Removing scabs may also mean removing new skin growth. Allow the access site to heal on its own.

It is important to listen to your access. It is an amazing sound like no other. Over time, you will learn what is normal and what is not normal. When listening, you may notice a change in blood flow through your access. Affordable stethoscopes are available at medical supply stores or pharmacies. Your dialysis team should also listen to the access before and again after each treatment.

You should hear a "whooshing" sound when listening to a graft or fistula access. This sound is called a "Bruit." Placing a stethoscope over the access incision, you should hear the bruit clearly. Continue listening along the entire length of the access. The sound will fade as you move away from the access incision area. The sound fading as you move away from the access site is normal. Abnormal sounds may be a light sound or no sound at all. Move the stethoscope to find the sound. If there is a faint sound or no sound at all, this may indicate slowing or stoppage of blood flow. Call the dialysis center immediately.

You may also feel your access. In order to feel your access, use your fingers and with a very light touch, move your fingers over the access. You will feel the tube-like access and feel a slight vibration. The vibration is called a "Thrill."

Whether you have a graft or a fistula, you should be able to hear and feel it. Over time, you will know what is normal and what is not normal for you. If you do not hear it or feel it, or if it sounds or feels different, report any abnormalities to your medical team so they can address these concerns and discuss them with you.

With any access, whether it is a catheter, graft or a fistula you will need to handle it with care. Be aware at all times where that access. Other than for dialysis, never let anyone stick that arm with needles. Never let anyone take your blood pressure on that arm. You need to take caution with the access as this is your passport to life.

In the event the access becomes damaged and needs replacing, this can be done much the same way the damaged access was originally placed. However, you should know there are limited places on your body where the surgeon can place an access, and you may find you are running out of suitable access sites if you are not careful. So respect the access and do not abuse it. Accesses can last for many years if taken care of properly.

The accesses, whether it is a fistula or graft, will last for several years, however, abusing the access, even unintentionally can cause it to need replacing sooner.

Limiting or Finding New Activities

Limiting activities can be a challenge all its own. The dialysis staff is a great source for information on what to limit and what to avoid. They can help find new activities that can be just as rewarding.

Or if crafting is not for you, try a new hobby that interests you. Find things that are enjoyable to you and make the best of life by doing new things. Life is sometimes about Plan B, and how you handle things that change with Plan A.

Find a way to pass the time and enjoy life. Dialysis is not the end of life. It is your passport to life. So enjoy it in any way you can.

Your dialysis clinic can advise you on any activities you may need to limit or avoid altogether. If you have questions about a certain activity, consult the dialysis team for guidance. They have access to all of the information you may need when caring for your access.

BLOOD THINNERS AND DIALYSIS

Part of the dialysis treatment includes the use of a blood thinner. The use of blood thinners during dialysis enables the blood to pass through the arteries or tubing and the machine easier. It also lessens a patient's chances of clotting. It will not prevent clotting of the catheter, fistula or graft all of the time, but it does reduce the clotting of the catheter, fistula or graft.

Blood thinners may also cause easy bruising and bleeding that can be difficult to stop. Caution must be taken to avoid cuts or bruises. Even a light touch can sometimes lead to bruising. A scratch can cause bleeding that, when using blood thinners, can be more difficult to control.

Bruising

Bruising, or contusion, is caused when the vessels or capillaries become damaged and blood leaks under the skin. With blood thinners, a person may bruise much easier than a person not using blood thinners. Bruising is normal with dialysis and also commonly seen with older people, even those not on dialysis or those not using blood thinners. With age, the skin becomes thinner and when coupled with thinning blood, it can cause bruising from something as simple as a light touch.

Do not be alarmed, but always communicate any bruising or cuts to the dialysis staff. Adjustments may be able to be made to lessen bruising or excessive bleeding. Always share any concerns you may have with the dialysis staff or medical staff.

If you experience bleeding or bruising, it is important to discuss this with your dialysis team. They may be able to adjust your treatment or amount of blood thinner to lessen bleeding or bruising.

You may also feel colder than usual. Remember, the blood is chilled during dialysis, so a certain amount of feeling cold is to be expected.

During dialysis, cover with a light blanket to stay warm leaving the access exposed allowing the staff to view it during treatment. Blood thinner and dialysis will both cause you to feel cold.

Bleeding

A person using blood thinning medication may find that bleeding from what seems like a simple scratch may be harder to control. Bleeding causes a loss of blood in the body that, in large amounts can be fatal. Access sites may bleed after dialysis. A small amount of blood is normal after a dialysis treatment. However, if you notice bleeding from the site at other times call or return to the dialysis center or call 911 immediately. If bleeding is excessive, call 911 immediately. Apply pressure to the site to slow or stop the bleeding as best you can until help arrives.

Blood thinners cause the blood to be thinner, hence the term 'blood thinner.' With thinner blood, the blood will not clot in a normal way, which can cause the body to continue to bleed. A person who does not use blood thinners and experiencing the cut may clot, and the bleeding is more controllable. Do not panic, light bleeding is normal although excessive bleeding requires immediate attention.

Never pick at the access sites. Scabs will likely form, but it is important never to pick at them as this may cause bleeding. Pulling off a scab may also pull out any clot that is preventing the site from bleeding. Scabs are also allowing for new skin growth and pulling a scab will also remove the new skin.

Remember blood thinners are being used to prevent clotting of the dialyzer.

Those patients who experience heart or blood disorders may use other forms of blood thinners. Your dialysis staff can assist you in what is best for you. Use extra caution when using blood thinners to avoid cuts or scratches.

Always follow the instructions of the dialysis staff and your doctors. They have the experience and the knowledge about your personal health information and can make more informed decisions about what is best for you.

If you have any questions about blood thinners or health care related questions, please direct them toward your dialysis staff or other healthcare professional.

Blood thinners can help with dialysis, but as with any medication, it can have side effects. Bleeding and bruising easily are two of the side effects.

So remember when you are taking blood thinners, which are a part of most dialysis treatments, be aware of your surroundings and take greater care not to scrape or cut yourself.

In the event you bleed, apply pressure to stop the bleeding. Once the bleeding is under control, call the dialysis clinic or 911 for assistance, if needed.

After each treatment, once the needles are removed, you will be asked to wait for a period of time, usually about 10 minutes to make certain bleeding has stopped. However, there are times when the bleeding can start again once you have left the clinic. If this happens, return to the clinic if possible and safe, or call 911. Remember to apply pressure to the area to control the bleeding.

RECOVERY PERIOD

After each dialysis treatment, a patient will need a period of time to recover from the treatment. The dialysis treatment removes and filters the blood from the body after which it then returns the cleansed blood to the body. It can be exhausting. It is necessary for a patient to rest afterward to allow the body to adjust to the changes in the body. It is a period that can range from an hour to several hours.

You may recover quicker or slower than others. The time it takes for recovery is a personal matter and based on how you feel after each treatment. It is a matter of how your body reacts to the treatment on that particular day. How you feel may mean not planning ahead for any activities on dialysis days after treatment.

You will have to make your own decisions as to what your limitations are and how much you can or cannot do or want or not want to do after treatment. No one else can, nor should they, expect you do more than you can do without first consulting with you.

If you were to think of what your body has been through, it only makes sense for a person to allow their body to readjust to the changes before you go about sometimes even minor activities. You may sleep for several hours while others can rest for an hour or more and recover fully. Some of this is age, and some has to do with other health issues you may have or perhaps just that day's treatment. Older patients may have a more difficult time recovering as quickly as a younger patient. A person with multiple health issues may find it more difficult to recover as quickly as a person with less health issues. By listening to your body, you will be able to make better decisions regarding your health. Only you, with your health care team's guidance, can make these decisions.

Your recovery period may not be the same amount of time after each treatment. It is important to remember this when making plans. Knowing how your body reacts to dialysis may be by trial and error that you, yourself, will need to learn. And through this process, you will know how much you can and cannot do after dialysis treatment. Do not let others make those decisions for you. You are the one who will suffer any consequences.

A general rule is not to plan anything other than treatment for dialysis days. Schedule appointments or other activities during the days you do not have a treatment. For instance, if you are a Monday, Wednesday and Friday dialysis patient, whenever possible, schedule doctor appointments and other activities for Tuesdays, Thursdays, Saturdays or Sundays. If you are a Tuesday, Thursday and Saturday dialysis patient whenever possible schedule doctor appointments and other activities only on Mondays, Wednesdays, Fridays or Sundays. While this is not always possible, it is best to not schedule appointments or activities on the same day you have dialysis whenever you can avoid doing so.

The treatment itself generally lasts four hours, when adding for time to connect and disconnect, getting to and from dialysis and a recovery period, which can be any amount of time, dialysis can be a full day.

If you need to be in the hospital, the hospital will arrange for dialysis treatments so you will not miss treatments during your stay in the hospital. Many hospitals now offer a small dialysis clinic area for temporary patients, although they may not offer permanent dialysis. They will be able to access or collect information regarding your dialysis treatments from your home dialysis center to assist them with your treatment.

Assisted living centers, nursing homes and other senior living centers may offer dialysis as well. If you are in need of those types of living arrangements, it may be available in your area.

Listen to your body and speak up. If you do not feel up to doing something, speak up and do what is best for you. Only you and no one else will suffer the consequences if you overdo it.

It is your body and only you know how it acts and reacts. It is important that you listen to what your body is telling you and to act on those changes. The dialysis staff can help you if you tell them of any changes in your body. They can assist in making it easier to adjust but only if you share that information with them. They cannot help if they do not know.

When first starting treatments, you will make adjustments and they will become the new normal for you. You will learn how to act and react to these changes as time goes on. Never take changes for granted until you learn the new normal and feel comfortable and know what to do in each situation. In time, the new normal will become routine.

Once you have been on dialysis for a while you will learn how much you can do after a treatment and when you will need to rest. Feeling tired is the body's way of saying slow down, take a break and rest. This is normal. No one can go without sleep or rest as it is a time for the body to rest. Take the time you need after a treatment to get rested so that you can enjoy the rest of the day. Take a break when you need it, you deserve it. Prior to dialysis treatments, you rested as needed, do the same now that you have started treatments as well. Do not overdo it. Take a rest and enjoy life.

If you have questions or concerns, talk to the dialysis staff. When in doubt, give a shout.

WHEN THINGS GO WRONG

Some believe they may live under what has become known as "Murphy's Law" where it is said, "If anything can go wrong, it will." Your health is certainly not immune from that "law." When things go wrong, the first thing to remember is to stay calm and not to be alarmed. Most things that go wrong may be more of a matter of the unknown. Not knowing is often worse than the situation once you know how to fix it or know that someone else knows how to fix the problem. You have to trust that your dialysis staff and your nephrology team know how to fix the glitches.

When you first begin dialysis, it is important to take notice of the changes in your body. No one knows your body better than you. We each have normal aches and pains, and we know when they are not 'normal' for us. At first you will notice many changes that you may believe are normal for dialysis patients. Although you may believe they are normal, do not take this as a reason not to share your concerns nor should you try to convince yourself that everything is normal. You need to know which is normal and which is not and this takes time after starting dialysis. Some things may be normal, and some may be abnormal. Changes may be made to accommodate for those changes.

Once your body and you adjust to these changes, you will learn that which is the new normal and that which is not. It does not mean things will be perfect but, over time, you will learn to adjust and know how to deal with the "new" normal you.

First, you need to know that the kidneys failing mean the body has likely not been functioning correctly for some time and dialysis will remove not only fluids but also the toxins that have built up in your body over time. Removing all of those toxins will likely take several treatments.

Many people believe that if they are not feeling bad that they do not need dialysis. Feeling good or bad is not an indication you need or do not need dialysis. Your treatments remove fluids, which, if not removed, can cause congestive heart failure and can be fatal. But dialysis also removes toxins that build up with kidney failure and so you need to make it to each treatment and always stay the entire time of your scheduled treatment. The more times a patient misses treatments, the more wear and tear on a patient's organs. Missing treatments can also cause more numbing and higher mortality rate.

If you can imagine the heart in a confined area, it needs room to expand as blood pushes through the heart supplying it to the various parts of the body, or we know it as heart pumping. As fluids build up in the body, it can build up around the heart as well as other more noticeable places, such as ankles and hands. When fluid builds up around the heart, the heart struggles to expand as needed because the fluids and heart compete for the same space. The heart can then fail to pump blood in sufficient amounts to the organs that rely on it to work properly. When this happens, it is called congestive heart failure. If the blood is not reaching the vital organs of the body that rely on it to feed them, it can cause those organs to not function.

Kidneys remove fluids through urination. A person also loses fluids through perspiration. When the kidneys fail, fluid is retained within the body. One of the purposes of dialysis is to remove the fluids that build up in the body. Removing these fluids allow the heart the room it needs to pump blood without that resistance. The organs are fed, the heart is not struggling and your life is much better.

You may notice a change in the area around your access. For instance a change in skin color or bumps are not normal, and you will need to contact someone to advise them of the changes. Bruising may be normal for some people who bruise easily, but redness, or abnormal color changes need to be addressed.

The first dialysis treatment will not likely be sufficient to remove enough of the toxins or even all of the fluid built up prior to any dialysis. Removing the toxins can take several treatments and even several months to reach a point of adjusting to the changes and your body feeling good again. It is not a lost cause just remember that when you start dialysis you will feel changes before you may begin to feel much better than you did prior to dialysis. Be patient and before long you will begin to feel much better.

Missing treatments means allowing more fluid and toxins to build up which can cause serious life-threatening conditions. So never, ever miss a treatment or sign out early just because you feel good that day. If you have to sign out before completing a treatment or if you miss a whole treatment, ask your dialysis center about scheduling an appointment time to make up that treatment the following day.

Over the many years since dialysis has been available, there have been patients somewhere who have encountered virtually every possible problem that can go wrong and there has been someone else who has found a solution to each of those problems. Do not panic. It is a matter of going to or calling the dialysis center and they will know what to do to fix the problem.

It is not an easy thing to stay calm when you are experiencing a problem with your access, but it is important to try and stay calm and get help immediately. Do not let problems go until your next treatment, call the dialysis center and inquire about whatever your concerns are. Once you have experienced more kidney failure symptoms, you will learn to recognize them and will learn which are normal and which need more immediate attention.

If the access is bleeding, and you cannot get it to stop within a minute or two, call 911 immediately.

Most of the problems may seem greater than they are, but the network of dedicated people who can help in virtually every situation is amazing. What may seem like a major thing to one person is a matter of knowing how to fix the problem to another. Keep them informed about changes you are experiencing and they can help you through it. If you do not tell them, they likely will not know.

It is also important that you, as a patient, learn all you can about the different aspects of your access and learn all you can about dialysis and even re-learn your body.

In the event that you find yourself in the emergency room, remembering things about your treatments can be helpful. Something as simple as remembering how much fluid they pulled off during the last treatment or even your weight after the last treatment or your dry weight can be useful information.

Understand that the emergency room staff is well trained in a lot of areas of health care but the training about dialysis will not likely compare to the same in depth type as that which the dialysis staff receives. Emergency room staffs may know some things about renal failure or different accesses, and some will seem to know more than others, but they will need help in determining what brought you to them. The problem may be another medical problem and unrelated to the dialysis however the body is a complicated piece of machinery, and they will need to know about the dialysis and any access you have among other things. All of this can assist the emergency room staff treat you.

Remember to never let others take blood pressure or use the dialysis arm for anything besides dialysis treatment. The access arm is always to be reserved for dialysis. Some accesses can easily be damaged and would require placement of another access. A person sticking you may easily damage the fistula or graft if not stuck correctly, so avoid anyone using that arm for anything other than dialysis. Ask them to place a "No Stick Right Arm" sign near you in the emergency or hospital bed if your access is in the right arm. Naturally this would be a left arm sign if your access is in the left arm. Access sites are limited and replacing too many different accesses may cause a person to run out of places to place them and cause some concern about how to treat the kidney failure.

Some of the things that can go wrong are easy to remedy and are also easy to prevent. For instance, if a patient is on overload of fluids, where they have drunk too many fluids between treatments, an additional dialysis treatment may help in remedying the problem they are experiencing. Fluid overload is caused by drinking excessive amounts of fluids. This can especially be true in summer or warmer temperatures. Try freezing grapes. In warm temperatures, sucking on a frozen grape will cool a person down and not add as much to the fluid intake say as a glass of water. Beware that a grape will not prevent heat exhaustion. You need to stay out of extremely hot environments to avoid dehydration and the need for additional fluids.

In other cases, it may mean the access has clotted, in which case, you will likely need a vascular surgeon or an interventionalist that can de-clot the access or they may decide you may need a new access. The medical team will determine that at the interventionalist or surgeon's office. Not all areas have interventionalists, and you may visit a vascular surgeon or even in many cases a general surgeon in areas where a vascular surgeon is not available to assist you.

You may not always know when to seek help or when you may need to go to an emergency room. A person knows their body better than anyone, and you will experience many changes during the first months of dialysis as your body adjusts to the changes. Once you have had time to adjust to the changes, you will relearn your body and will know when to seek help. Never hesitate to communicate with your dialysis staff, nephrologist or other medical teams about any questions or concerns you may have. If you feel chest pain, light headed, have bleeding or just overall not feeling well before or after after treatment, call 911 immediately. If you have any of these symptoms during a treatment, you should immediately alert the dialysis staff. These can be serious symptoms, and you need to seek immediate medical help. Do not wait until the next treatment date. You may also call your dialysis center if it is not life threatening.

With dialysis, there may be some nausea, constipation, drop in blood pressure and dizziness. If you experience any of these symptoms while on the dialysis machine, you should alert the staff immediately. You may also have bleeding from the site after dialysis. Apply pressure and stop the bleeding. If you are unable to stop the bleeding, return to the dialysis center or call 911 immediately noting that the bleeding is not stopping. Tell them you are a dialysis patient and have bleeding from the access site allowing them to expedite help.

Other complications may be overall not feeling well. This is to be expected with starting dialysis until the body adjusts to the treatments and changes the treatments are causing in your body. Talk to the dialysis staff about all of these changes until you learn which are normal and which need attention.

There are many things that can go wrong or seem to be just not right when you are taking dialysis. You will find your body changes, and you will need to adjust to those changes.

Once you have been on dialysis for a while, you will know how your body feels at each point, and you will know more about how to handle each of those feelings. Always, always, always talk to the dialysis staff about the differences you may be experiencing. It may be something minor, or they may be able to adjust the treatment to fine-tune it to your needs. Never assume that it is just the way it is and not speak up. Even the slightest difference may be able to be lessened, or there may be something they or someone else can do to make you more comfortable.

Never assume anything. Until you understand all of the changes, it is best to speak up. After you understand the changes, you should still speak up. Let them know what is bothering you and how you feel. If you do not, they may never know.

Common problems can be when the access narrows, or stenosis. It is not uncommon for the graft or fistula to narrow after extended use. The dialysis clinic should know if it is narrowing by your intra-access flow rate. If you have reduced flow rate, the alarm will sound on the machine, and it is a distinct sound to alert the staff of the problem.

Another common problem is clotting of the blood, or thrombosis, in the veins, which can usually be de-clotted by the nephrologist or interventionalist. A de-clot, as it is sometimes called, is a procedure used to open a fistula or graft. A nephrologist, or interventionalist, inserts a tiny balloon into the access, blowing up the balloon allowing the vein to stretch and pop the vein open allowing the clot to be removed. At times, you can hear the popping sound. Once this is done, the access should be free of the clot, and you may continue using the access for your dialysis treatments as directed by the nephrologist or interventionalist. In the event you cannot use the access immediately, the nephrologist or vascular surgeon can likely insert a catheter to use until the access site is once again ready to be used.

Another common problem is aneurysms. An aneurysm is when the vein or graft bulges. The bulge can be noticeable and the larger it gets, the more concerned a person may be. If the skin becomes thin or shiny, it can be a sign that the access can be at risk of bursting. This can also be true of a graft and can be a sign of a breakdown of the walls of the graft.

Infections are of concern as well. With the access site being an access to the blood stream, infections are always a concern. Bacteria entering the blood stream are always a possibility when there are open accesses to the bloodstream. It is extremely important to take care of the access site and to report any concern to the staff, no matter how small it may seem. A sign of infection is when the access site is red, or discolored. Bruising may be normal for some on dialysis. A dialysis patient is given blood thinners and can bruise easily. To protect the access, always keep it covered and clean it often.

If the site is draining pus or abnormally sore, alert someone immediately as this can be a sign of infection or thrombosis.

Wear loose clothing over the site area and do not allow tight jewelry to obstruct that area that can cause the site to narrow.

DIALYSIS AND DIET

Understanding the Dialysis Diet

Once you begin dialysis treatments, the diet you may have once known and followed will change. You will now need to eat more high quality protein rich foods, while also consuming less sodium, potassium, phosphorus and liquids.

Later in this book, there is a recommended grocery list which will help in the types of foods to eat and those to limit. But how do you know the amounts you can have of each? Food labels are not designed for a dialysis diet. Reading the labels can be confusing for a dialysis patient.

This chapter will try to help you understand the diet needed and how to determine if you are eating right to feel right. Of course, each dialysis center has a dietitian available and you can direct any questions or concerns to them and they are able to help in your own dietary needs.

Each patient is different and not all patients can eat each food, or may just not like that food, and so a dietitian can help create a menu that is best for you. Always take advantage of the help that is available to you. There are vast resources available if you have a need and any question can be answered and make living with renal failure easier.

Changes to Your Diet

We all understand that diet is important even before dialysis. But now that your kidneys no longer work the way that they should, a new diet along with your dialysis treatments will help keep extra water and waste from building up in your body.

You will need to limit foods that are high in

Sodium

Sodium can be found in foods in natural forms. For instance, seafood can be naturally high in sodium. Sodium can also be found in processed foods. Preservatives used in foods can contain high amounts of sodium. Salty foods are, of course, high in sodium. Sodium can cause the body retain fluids as well as cause you to be thirsty, and it can raise blood pressure. Limiting sodium does not mean eating a bland diet.

It is found in large amounts in table salt and in many other foods. You may find foods without added salt are bland but in time, you will adjust to these new flavors and learn to use certain herbs and spices to make your food taste good. After all, we eat for tastes and a bland diet is hard to swallow sometimes.

You will need to avoid some foods that are known to be high in sodium such as:

Most canned foods and some frozen dinners,

Processed meats like hot dogs, bacon & cold cuts

Canned and dry soup mixes, canned vegetables

Condiments such as BBQ sauce, soy sauce, mustard, relish, ketchup, onion salt, garlic salt, seasoning salt. Even those products that are no salt or low sodium may contain higher levels of potassium.

Many processed foods contain sodium based preservatives and will need to be avoided.

Potassium

Potassium is another important mineral found in food. Potassium is a mineral that's crucial for life. It makes your muscles and heart work properly. It is likely that you will need to limit the amount of high-potassium food. You eat each day. Potassium is necessary for the heart, kidneys, and other organs to work normally. High levels of potassium can be found in bananas, beans and potatoes to name a few. It is also found in halibut, salmon and tuna. Potassium is removed during the dialysis treatment although you will need to limit the amounts between treatments.

Large amounts of potassium are found in foods such as:

Bananas, cantaloupe or honeydew melon, oranges

Fruits such as raisins, apricots, prunes and dates

Potatoes*, tomatoes, squash, spinach

Orange juice, prune juice, tomato juice and vegetable juice.

Milk, cheese and yogurt

Most salt substitutes (check with your doctor or dietitian before using)
Chocolate, coffee, nuts, dried beans, split peas

Bran cereal, whole wheat foods

*Potatoes can be treated to can reduce potassium by up to 80% making them suitable for dialysis patient diet. The process is simple, though time consuming.

Wash and peel potatoes. Cut potatoes into pieces. Soak them in room temperature water for 5 hours. Drain and rinse the potatoes. Repeat the process in fresh room temperature water for additional 2 hours. Drain and rinse the potatoes and prepare as you normally would. This process is said to remove up to 80% of the potassium in the potatoes and can make them safer for renal patients to enjoy potatoes once again. If you are a meat and potato kind of person, here is a healthy alternative to allow you to enjoy potatoes once again.

You will find that before a procedure to insert access, a blood test will be preformed to look at potassium levels. The potassium level is crucial to determining when a patient needs treatment. High levels of potassium can cause complications. Complications can include arrhythmia (heart rhythm problems). It will be determined prior to the procedure if a patient will need a treatment immediately following the procedure.

Phosphorus

Phosphorus is an important element in the body. It helps to regulate the calcium which makes teeth and bones strong. It is not unusual for dialysis patients to later have brittle bones from low phosphorus levels.

You will receive a prescription for binders once you begin dialysis treatments. The binder is used with each meal to capture the phosphorus and bind it to the solid waste which is then removed with a bowel movement. The number of binders taken is determined by your phosphorus levels. If you know you are eating foods that may be high in phosphorus, your dialysis staff may tell you to take extra binders. This is not a free pass to eat uncontrollable amounts of phosphorus and the diet should be followed as much as you are able to.

Some foods high in phosphorus are milk, cheese and beans. Alternatives are available and should be used whenever possible. For instance, instead of a ½ cup of ice cream with 80 grams of phosphorus, try a ½ cup of sherbet or a Popsicle with 0 grams of phosphorus, but remember that ice cream, sherbet and a Popsicle count as liquid. Any food that is liquid at room temperature will count as a liquid. You need to avoid too many liquids.

Eating foods high in phosphorus will raise the phosphorus level in your blood and over time, it will weaken your bones. It is important to limit the amount of high phosphorus foods in your diet. Phosphorus is a mineral that is found in large amounts in foods such as:

Dairy products such as milk, cheese, yogurt, ice cream

Nuts and peanut butter

Dried beans and peas such as kidney beans, split peas and lentils

Beverages such as cocoa, beer and dark cola drinks

Liquids

Once starting dialysis, liquids will become limited. The dialysis machine takes off the excess fluids. However, the excess fluids can build up between treatments and cause complications such as bloating, swollen ankles and feet, and can cause congestive heart failure. This is discussed elsewhere in this book, but if the heart is constricted by fluids around the heart, or the lungs can be restricted by fluid building up, they cannot operate as needed to provide the body with blood or oxygen. Lack of blood or oxygen to vital parts of the body will cause complications and even death.

Drinking too many liquids may cause you to become short of breath, have swelling in your legs or have high blood pressure. Your dietitian will help you understand what the safe amount of liquid is for you each day.

Liquids (fluids) are foods or beverages that are liquid at room temperature, such as:

Coffee, tea

Sodas, Sport drinks, juice, lemonade, beer, wine

Ice, Popsicle, sherbet, ice cream and gelatin

Soup and broth

Water, ice cubes

To keep track of all of the liquid that you drink each day, use a measuring cup to find out the amount of liquid that your favorite glass and mug hold. Until you get used to measuring, keep track of the amount of liquid you drink each day on a sheet of paper or notebook.

Protein

Your diet will need to include more high quality protein foods like lean meat, egg whites (egg whites contain high quality protein while egg yellows or yolks are high in cholesterol), egg substitutes, fish, pork, seafood (being careful of sodium levels in some seafood), and poultry to meet your daily protein needs.

The body needs protein to allow the body to grow and to make nails, hair and skin healthy. It also can be dangerous if a person has too much protein. Too much protein can cause the kidneys to work harder and this can cause the kidneys to break down or fail sooner. While the two main causes of kidney failure have been linked to high blood pressure and diabetes, protein can also be a factor in kidney function.

Changing the protein part of the diet to a high quality protein can help with staying healthier. It is recommended that you talk to your dietitian for more information. They can offer advice on how to maintain a healthy level of protein.

Some protein-rich foods may also contain a lot of phosphorus, a mineral you now need to limit in your diet.

Your dietitian will help you plan a diet with the right amount of protein for your good health and strength.

Renal Dietitians

Renal dietitians are a great source of information about the renal diet. They are specially trained in renal diets and can help with your questions. They can also help you with a shopping list, cooking ideas, meal planning and even which restaurants have renal friendly meals.

The dietitians are well trained and can help you in many ways with diet and do's and do not's of dialysis. They are there for a reason and you are encouraged to use their knowledge to help you.

Following a special diet can be fun and healthy for you. It can broaden your food experiences and you will find new flavors that you would not have explored if it were not for the need to change diets.

Renal Diet

While the renal diet, in many ways can be restrictive, it can also be fun and exciting to try new combinations of foods, herbs and spices. We all get set on a certain menu and feel we just cannot live without a certain food or drink. It is not until we are sometimes forced to make a change that we realize we have been missing a world of new flavors. Be daring and try new things. Eat to live instead of living to eat.

We all eat for taste and you can still do that, but change the herbs and spices to make you healthier. Explore the possibilities and you may be surprised at what you may find.

The dialysis diet is not so restrictive that you cannot enjoy food. You need only make changes to the diet to align with what is best for you now that you are on dialysis.

In this book, you will see a list entitled the "Suggested Grocery List." That list is not all of the foods you can eat, your dietitian can help make a more detailed list based on your own needs, but the list has a lot of foods you are already familiar with. Change the diet to those foods and remember to stick to your diet and you will fare better.

Breakdown of Diet

How do you know how much liquid, potassium, phosphorus and sodium is acceptable and how much is too much?

Daily intake of liquids may be limited. Many patients are limited to one liter a day. Your dietitian can tell you how much you need to limit yourself to. One of the factors in determining amount of fluids allowed might be whether or not you are still urinating. Some people with renal failure urinate less than before and some do not urinate at all. If the body is still emptying the bladder, your fluid levels may be different than a person who does not urinate and therefore retains the fluids.

The amount of daily potassium will also be limited for those on dialysis. Most dialysis patients will need to limit their daily potassium intake to 2000 to 3000 milligrams. Your dietitian can help you set the level you may need. Peritoneal patients may be allowed higher amounts.

Phosphorus will be limited. You may be limited to 800 to 1000 milligrams of phosphorus per day. Of course, binders will help reduce phosphorus retained in the body. Your doctor or nurse can assist you with binder control. Sometimes, when phosphorus is raised, or you eat foods on occasion that may be a little high in phosphorus, you can take an extra binder to offset any additional phosphorus. The doctor may also be able to prescribe a different binder if you are over on the phosphorus levels. Do not take that to be a free ride to ignore the diet. While the binders can help offset changes, a well followed diet is still best.

Sodium can help the body retain water and make the kidneys work harder. Sodium will be limited by not adding salt to foods and eating those foods that are low in sodium naturally as described above.

Sodium is found in many foods and a careful watch needs to be made for sodium levels in foods.

Protein will need to be increased for most people. A rule might be to eat 0.8 grams of protein for each kilogram of your body weight. A kilogram is about 2.2 pounds. For instance if you weigh 60kg, or 150 pounds, your daily intake of protein may be 120 grams of protein or about 4.5 ounces of high quality protein per day.

With all of these suggestions, you are advised to talk to your dietitian and allow them to set your limits on each of these and allow them to use their knowledge to help you live better.

A renal diet is not that hard to adjust to if you are willing to change some simple things about your diet.

People do not usually like changes but if you are willing to experiment with the diet and try new types of foods, or even old favorites with a new twist, you may find it is a wonderful change for you. Be adventurous and dare to try something different. And be thankful you are not in a county where they eat bugs for survival. The diet is full of options and being creative can be fun and rewarding.

If you or someone you know, like to cook, this is an amazing opportunity for the cooking creations to fly out. A person who likes to cook may see this as a challenge and who can resist a challenge?

Make a choice to eat healthier and have fun.

SUGGESTED GROCERY LIST
(Reprinted with reprint permission of Abbot Laboratories)

Meat/High Protein Foods

Beef
Chicken
Egg Substitute (Egg Beaters®, Scramblers®)
Eggs
Fish
Lamb
Pork (fresh)
 (Pork chops, roast)
Shellfish
Tofu (soft)
Tuna (canned in water)
Turkey
Veal
Wild Game

Fruits
(Serving Size = 1 medium size fruit or 1/2 cup canned, no added sugar)

Apple Juice
Apples
Apple Sauce
Apricot nectar
Apricots (canned)
Blackberries
Cherries
Cranberries
Cranberry Juice
Figs (fresh)
Fruit Cocktail

Grapefruit
Grape Juice
Grapes
Lemon
Lemon Juice
Lime
Lime Juice
Loganberries
Lychees
Peach (canned)
Peach nectar
Pears (canned)
Pineapple
Plums
Raspberries
Strawberries
Tangerines

Vegetables
(Serving Size – 1/2 cup, no added salt)

Alfalfa Sprouts
Arugula
Asparagus
Bean Sprouts
Beets (canned)
Cabbage (green, red)
Carrots
Cauliflower
Celery
Chayote
Chili Peppers
Chives

Coleslaw
Corn
Cucumber
Eggplant
Endive
Garlic
Gingerroot
Green Beans
Hominy
Jalapeños
Kale
Leeks
Lettuce
Mixed Vegetables
Mushrooms
Onions
Parsley
Peas (English)
Pimentos
Radicchio
Radishes
Seaweed kelp
Spaghetti Squash
Summer Squash (scallop, crookneck, straightneck, zucchini)
Sweet Peppers (Green, Yellow, Red)
Tomatillos
Turnips
Turnip Greens
Water Chestnuts
Watercress
Yam bean (jicama), cooked

Breads/Cereals/Grain

Bagels (plain, blueberry, egg, raisin)
Bread (white, French, Italian, rye, soft wheat)
Bread sticks (plain)
Cereals, dry, low salt (Corn Pops®, Cocoa Puffs®, Sugar Smacks®, Fruity Pebbles®, Puffed Wheat®, Puffed Rice®)
Cereals, cooked (Cream of Wheat®, or Wheat Farina®, Malt-o-Meal®)
Crackers (unsalted)
Dinner rolls or hard rolls
English muffins
Grits
Hamburger/hot dog buns
Macaroni
Melba toast
Noodles
Oyster crackers
Pita bread
Popcorn (unsalted)
Pretzels (unsalted)
Rice (brown, white)
Rice cakes (apple-cinnamon, etc.)
Spaghetti
Tortillas

Dairy/Dairy Substitutes

Nondairy frozen desserts (Mocha Mix®)
Rice milk, unfortified
Nondairy frozen dessert topping (Cool Whip®)

Nondairy creamers

Beverages

(Keep in mind you fluid restriction) (Diabetics – use caution for sugar intake) (Regular or Diet)

7-Up®
Cherry 7-Up®
Cream soda
Ginger ale
Grape soda
Lemon-lime soda
Mellow-Yellow®
Mountain Dew®
Orange soda
Root beer
Slice®
Sprite®
Coffee
Fruit
Hi-C® (Cherry, grape)
Horchata®
Juices (apple, cranberry, grape)
Kool-Aid®
Lemonade or Limeade
Mineral water
Nectars (apricot, peach, pear, 1/2 cup serving)
Nondairy creamers (Coffee Rich®, Mocha Mix®, etc.)
Sunny Delight® (citrus flavor)
Tea

Fats

Butter
Cream Cheese
Margarine
Mayonnaise
Miracle Whip®
Nondairy creamers
Salad dressings
Sour cream
Vegetable oils (preferably canola or olive oil)

Seasonings and Spices

Allspice
Basil
Bay Leaf
Caraway
Chives
Cilantro
Cinnamon
Cloves
Cumin
Curry
Dill
Extracts (almond, lemon, lime, maple, orange, peppermint, vanilla, walnut)
Fennel
Garlic powder
Ginger
Horseradish (root)
Lemon Juice

Mrs. Dash®
Nutmeg
Onion powder or flakes
Oregano
Paprika
Parsley or parsley flakes
Pepper (ground)
Pimentos
Poppy seed
Rosemary
Saccharin
Saffron
Sage
Savory
Sesame seeds
Tarragon
Thyme
Turmeric
Vinegar

Desserts/Snacks/Sweets
(Diabetics Use Caution)

Animal crackers
Cake (angel food, butter, lemon, pound, spice, strawberry, white, yellow)
Candy corn
Chewing gum
Cinnamon drops
Cookies (ginger snaps, shortbread, sugar, vanilla wafers)

Corn cakes
Cotton Candy
Doughnuts
Fruit ice
Graham crackers
Gumdrops
Gummy Bears®
Hard candy
Hot Tamale® candy
Jell-O®
Jelly beans
Jolly Rancher®
Life Savers®
Lollipops
Marshmallows
Newton's® (fig, strawberry, apple, blueberry)
Pie (apple, berry, cherry, lemon, peach)

Other
(Diabetics - Use Caution)

Apple Butter
Corn syrup
Honey
Jam
Jelly
Maple Syrup
Marmalade
Powdered sugar
Sugar, brown or white

FREQUENTLY ASKED QUESTIONS (FAQ)

In this section, we will look at various questions you may have. In some instances, the answers may be found elsewhere in this book in more detail. This information is provided solely for informational purposes and is not to be considered medical advice, nor as a substitute for medical care. If you have any questions, please refer them to a qualified medical professional.

What are the kidneys and what do they do?

The kidneys are two bean-shaped organs, each about the size of a fist. They are located just below the rib cage, one on each side of the spine. Every day, the two kidneys filter about 120 to 150 quarts of blood to produce about 1 to 2 quarts of urine, composed of wastes and extra fluid. The urine flows from the kidneys to the bladder through two thin tubes of muscle called ureters, one on each side of the bladder. The bladder stores urine. The muscles of the bladder wall remain relaxed while the bladder fills with urine. As the bladder fills to capacity, signals sent to the brain tell a person to empty their bladder. When the bladder empties, urine flows out of the body through a tube called the urethra, located at the bottom of the bladder.

Why are the kidneys important?

The kidneys are important because they keep the composition, or makeup, of the blood stable, which lets the body function. They:
- prevent the buildup of wastes and extra fluid in the body,
- keep levels of electrolytes stable, such as sodium, potassium, and phosphate,
- make hormones that help :
  - regulate blood pressure,
  - make red blood cells,
  - Bones stay strong.

Why do I need dialysis?

The kidneys are considered one of the seven vital organs of the human body. If a person's kidneys fail to function at an adequate level to remove wastes or produce urine, dialysis is needed to perform those functions. If a person does not receive dialysis, the life expectancy of that person is limited to the amount of time it will take for fluid and wastes to build up within the body. The amount of time a person may survive without the use of their kidneys or dialysis varies slightly but can be less than 45 days. The amount of time varies depending on the level of kidney function and amounts of toxins or fluids that are built up within the body.

If I have a catheter for dialysis, why do I need a graft or a fistula also?

The catheter is a temporary access that is used until a more permanent access, such as a graft or fistula, matures. Catheters are not meant to be used long-term. Catheters have a higher risk of causing infection and increased mortality. Also, a catheter can attach itself to the artery, and this can cause complications when removing the catheter. While waiting for the fistula or graft to mature (or heal), the catheter is a means to receive treatment. A graft or fistula can take weeks to mature. A patient in need of dialysis cannot afford to wait for weeks for the access to mature before receiving treatment. Remember, if a patient does not receive dialysis, the patient may only survive a short period. Therefore, a catheter is the first access a patient will receive though it is a temporary access and should be removed once a more permanent access is available.

Why did my kidneys stop working?

There are a number of reasons why kidneys fail. Two of the most common reasons kidneys fail are diabetes and uncontrolled high blood pressure (hypertension). While these are not the only reasons, they are the most common. Other reasons can include trauma to the body, such as an automobile accident. These are just a few of the reasons. To understand what may have caused your kidneys to fail, you will need to consult your medical professionals.

Will I need dialysis the rest of my life?

Most dialysis patients will need treatments for the remainder of their lives. However, this is not always the case. There are times when a dialysis patient may find their kidneys have returned to a greater level of functioning, and they may no longer need dialysis. This is referred to as acute renal function that was resolved. While this is rare, it does happen on occasion.

My kidneys have failed. What are my options?

When a person's kidneys fail, there are options available today. A kidney transplant is one option. However, that is a long term plan and not an immediate plan. It can take time to find a donor's kidney, and there is a waiting list for a kidney. In the meantime, patients are faced with dialysis.

There are different options for dialysis. The different types of dialysis are discussed in more detail in this book. However, they are in clinic dialysis, home dialysis or peritoneal dialysis. For a better understanding of your options, please consult with your medical professionals as each case is different. Your options will be determined by the clinic staff and nephrologist and they can decide the best course of action needed to meet your needs.

Why do I need a four-hour treatment? Can this be shortened?

The patient's individual needs determine the length of a patient's treatment. A longer treatment is better for the patient than a shorter treatment, even when those shorter treatments are more often. The blood needs to be cleaned, and fluids need to be removed. Pushing too much blood, too fast through the body causes the organs to work harder. Over time, shorter treatments can cause damage to organs including the heart. There is no such thing as too much dialysis, there are many complications with too little dialysis.

I have been on dialysis for a while, and I feel good. Do I still need dialysis?

If you feel good congratulations! Your dialysis is probably working well for you. But, dialysis is not only about feeling good. Dialysis is not a cure for kidney failure. Rather, it is a treatment to keep the blood cleansed and fluids removed with each treatment. In between treatments, your body will again build up toxins and fluids, requiring another treatment to remove those toxins and fluids before they reach a safe level. Failing to be treated on a regular basis allows the toxins and fluids to build up at levels that can be dangerous. A person with kidney failure needs regularly scheduled dialysis treatments to cleanse the blood and remove excess fluids. A person may feel good because of their treatments, and it is sometimes confused with not needing treatment because they feel good today. While feeling good is one of the goals of dialysis, it is not the only goal. Failing to be treated will lead to organs not functioning and many other complications. For instance, fluids can build up around the heart and lungs making it difficult to breathe. Missing treatments can also put a patient at risk for heart failure and arrhythmia which can lead to death if not treated. Each time a patient misses a treatment or signs out of treatment early, the toxins and fluids have an opportunity to build up to unhealthy levels.

Can I take a 12-hour treatment once a week instead of 4 hours a day, three days a week?

Unfortunately, the answer is no. As you take in food and liquids, the body needs to be cleaned to remove those fluids and toxins in the blood. Allowing the body a longer time to accumulate those fluids and toxins can cause the body to absorb more into the blood. The kidneys worked 24 hours a day. Dialysis limits the same process to that time a patient is being dialyzed. It is important to keep each dialysis appointment and not to sign out early from any treatment. It is imperative for the patient to stay on the dialysis machine to allow the machine to filter properly the blood and to do the job the kidneys can no longer do.

What is the difference between a nephrologist and an interventionalist?

A nephrologist is a medical doctor who specializes in kidneys. An interventionalist is a medical doctor who may be a nephrologist but has additional specialized training in solving problems with dialysis accesses. Some of the problems may be clotting of the fistula or graft. The interventionalist can perform a procedure to clear the fistula or graft of the clot. The interventionalist may also insert and remove catheters. These procedures may also be performed by a cardiovascular or general surgeon.

Why does my access clot?

The access is a channel for blood to flow through, much like a vein or artery. Clotting is a natural process within the body to prevent bleeding. Once the needles have been removed after a dialysis treatment the blood clots to prevent the site from bleeding. When this happens, you will be sent to a procedure center or surgeon to have the access de-clotted. This procedure is described earlier in this book.

I listened to my access, and I do not hear anything. Should I tell someone about this?

Whenever there is a change in the sound or feel of your access, it is always best to tell the dialysis staff or your doctor. The access might have become clotted, or it may be narrowing or slowing down. In this case, you will need to have it de-clotted or repaired to complete dialysis treatments.

My fingers on my access arm get numb. Is this normal?

Numbness and cold in the arm or hand could mean the blood is not flowing to those areas in sufficient amounts. It is similar to the hand or leg "going to sleep." Making a fist and releasing it several times may help to "wake up" the hand and restart the blood flow. This may also be a nerve issue. You will need to contact someone. As is the case with any concern a patient may have, do not hesitate to call someone with concerns. Remember, when in doubt, give a shout!!!

Why does my skin feel itchy after dialysis?

Most dialysis patients feel itchy at times. Many say it is worse after dialysis. A person who experiences itchiness after dialysis may have a high level of phosphorous in their system. A sample shopping list is found in this book, to include many low phosphorous foods. Patients are prescribed medication to assist in reducing phosphorous. These medications are referred to as binders and help reduce phosphorous which, as the name implies, binds the phosphorus that is then removed from the body through bowel movements.

Another cause of itchiness is allergies. Antihistamines can sometimes be taken for allergic reactions. Always consult a medical professional before taking any medication, even those available over the counter. Medications can have an adverse reaction with other medications. Your doctor will be able to advise you on this.

Dry skin may also cause the itchiness. Dialysis patients should avoid hot places, such as direct sunlight or long hot showers. Using a natural soap without chemicals and a lotion will help with dry skin. Apply the lotion right after a shower while the body is still warm and damp.

The needles they use for dialysis hurt my arm. Is there something I can do to limit the pain?

Yes. The nephrologist or dialysis staff can suggest or prescribe a numbing agent to patients who feel discomfort from the needles. It can be a spray or a cream that should be applied before dialysis. Also, they will be able to show you how to apply either to get the best results.

How long will my fistula last?

If a fistula is taken care of, it can last for decades. A fistula is a natural access created by connecting an artery and vein together and, therefore, can last a lifetime. Taking care of the fistula is important to maintain a healthy access.

Is the fistula or graft a better access type?

A fistula is the preferred type of access because it is a natural type. Placing a foreign object in the body can cause complications not found when using a person's natural arteries and veins. While a fistula is the preferred type of access, not all people can use their veins and a graft becomes necessary.

How do I know if my access site is infected?

Infections are a concern with dialysis patients. An infection can be a nuisance, or it can be life-threatening if left untreated. It is important to know the signs of infection and to report any concerns to the health care team to allow them to investigate. Infections may be noticeable if the access site is tender, red, swollen, irritated. Or drainage from the access site. A fever can also be a sign of infection. Because many dialysis patients are diabetic, there is a risk of infection when the glucose level is high for these patients.

If the access site should become infected, it may affect the ability to have dialysis. By having a treatment when an area is infected, it can introduce the infection to the bloodstream causing serious complications. If a patient feels they may have an infection, they are advised to alert the staff immediately so they can investigate and determine which course of action to take.

What happens if my graft stops working?

In the event the graft should stop working, there are a number of things that can be done. First, it needs to be determined why it stopped working. It may be a relatively simple de-clot. In which case, it would be a matter of opening the graft up again allowing blood to flow.

Another reason the graft may have stopped working could be that it has been pinched reducing or cutting off the flow of blood. The patient may need stents or angioplasty to correct the problem.

In other cases, the graft becomes worn and needs to be replaced. If this is the case, the patient will need a new vein mapping before a new graft can be placed.

After dialysis, I bleed from my access site. Is this normal?

Some bleeding is normal; however, before leaving the dialysis center, any bleeding should have stopped. Applying pressure to the access site for a period of time, usually about 5 to 10 minutes after dialysis, should be adequate to stop the bleeding.

The dialysis staff will not let a patient leave if the bleeding has not stopped. Once leaving the dialysis center, if bleeding begins again, apply pressure to the site and return to the dialysis center immediately or call 911 in the case of excess bleeding.

How do I listen to my access?

When listening to the access, it is best to use a device named a stethoscope. Place the stethoscope on top of the access area and gently move the stethoscope along the length of the access. A whooshing sound should be heard. If it is not heard, try re-positioning the stethoscope. By moving the stethoscope further away from the access point, the sound will begin to fade. This is normal. If a sound is not heard, call the dialysis center as the absence of sound may mean the access has stopped working.

What causes me to cramp during or shortly after dialysis?

Cramping is a common occurrence during or shortly after dialysis. Cramping can be caused by removing fluid at a fast rate or removing large amounts of fluid. Removing blood at a fast rate can cause the body to react by cramping. Ask the staff for advice on controlling the cramping.

Low potassium may also cause cramping. During dialysis, potassium is removed and the body may react by cramping.

Why does my blood pressure suddenly drop during dialysis?

Removing fluid may cause low blood pressure. Low blood pressure is a common side effect of dialysis. If a patient is taking blood pressure medication they should consult their doctor about possibly not taking that medication prior to a dialysis treatment. Always consult a doctor or other medical professional before changing medications or changing the routine of taking medications.

My access arm has a bump the size of a golf ball. Should I be concerned about this?

A bump on the access area may be an aneurysm. An aneurysm occurs when the wall of the fistula or graft has a weakened spot and the blood has entered the weak spot making a "bubble" in the fistula or graft. This can be problematic. Should an aneurysm leak or bust, it will bleed, which can cause a drop in blood pressure or even death if not repaired.

Another cause of a bump around the access may be what is known as infiltration. Infiltration occurs when the needle misses or slips outside of the fistula or graft during dialysis allowing blood to build up under the skin. If this occurs during dialysis, alert the dialysis staff immediately.

Anything that looks out of place needs to be addressed with a medical professional.

Can I travel with kidney failure? How will I get my treatments?

Dialysis patients can travel. Their local dialysis center can arrange for treatments along their route to enable them to receive treatments as they travel. By giving the local dialysis center a copy of the travel plans, or itinerary, they should be able to assist in arranging treatments in clinics along the way.

In fact, one dialysis patient rode a bicycle across the United States scheduling treatments on a regular schedule. While this may not be something each patient can do, or want to do, traveling is possible.

Home dialysis and peritoneal patients can take the machine and supplies with them and perform their treatments virtually anywhere, while in clinic dialysis patients will need to schedule treatments in a center near their route of travel or destination. A peritoneal dialysis patient can make arrangements to pick up supplies at dialysis centers across the United States and if the need arises, treatments can be arranged at a dialysis center.

If my access fails, will I still be able to get treatment?

Yes. If the access fails, the access can be repaired and treatment can resume. If the access can not be repaired and a new access is needed an alternative method of access can be established to allow treatments to be performed. A catheter can be inserted, similar to the one when you likely had previously.

GLOSSARY

A person who has been diagnosed with renal complications and their caregiver, will likely hear and read many new terms they may not have heard or read about previously. Below is a list of some of those terms.

NOTE: Information in this glossary is not a substitute for a visit to your doctor or professional advice. Do not attempt diagnose or treat yourself. Talk with a health professional if you have a problem with your kidney failure treatment.

A

access: In *dialysis*, the point on the body where the dialysis staff obtains a path to your blood. See *arteriovenous fistula*, *graft*, and *vascular access* and catheter.

arterial line (ar-TIHR-ee-uhl) (lyn): in *hemodialysis*, the tubing that takes blood from the body to the *dialyzer*. See *hemodialysis* under *dialysis*.

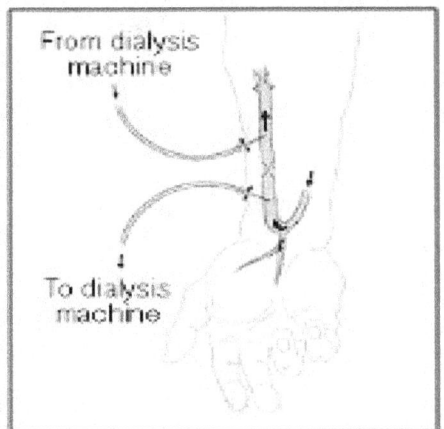

Arteriovenous fistula

arteriovenous (AV) fistula (ar-TIHR-ee-oh-VEE-nuhss) (FISS-tyoo-luh): surgical connection of an *artery* directly to a *vein*, usually in the forearm, created in people who will need *hemodialysis*. The AV fistula causes the vein to grow thicker, allowing the repeated needle insertions required for hemodialysis. Development of the AV fistula takes 4 to 8 weeks after surgery before it can be used for hemodialysis. The AV fistula is the preferred method of *access*. See *hemodialysis* under *dialysis*.

arteriovenous (AV) graft (ar-TIHR-ee-oh-VEE-nuhss) (graft): in *hemodialysis*, surgical connection of an *artery* to a *vein* using a soft, flexible tube, which can be used for repeated needle sticks. See *hemodialysis* under *dialysis*.

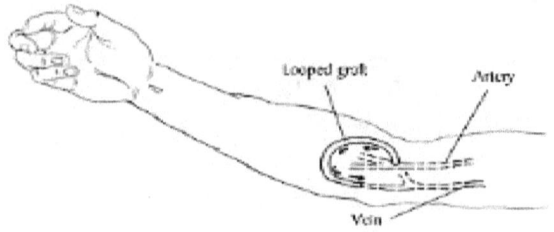

Arteriovenous Graft

artery (AR-tur-ee): a large blood vessel that carries blood with oxygen from the heart to all parts of the body.

C

CAPD (SEE-AY-PEE-DEE): see *continuous ambulatory peritoneal dialysis* under *dialysis*.

catheter (KATH-uh-tur): a tube inserted through the skin into a blood vessel or cavity to draw out body fluid or infuse fluid. In *peritoneal dialysis*, a catheter is used to infuse *dialysis solution* into the abdominal cavity and drain it out again. See *peritoneal dialysis* under *dialysis*.

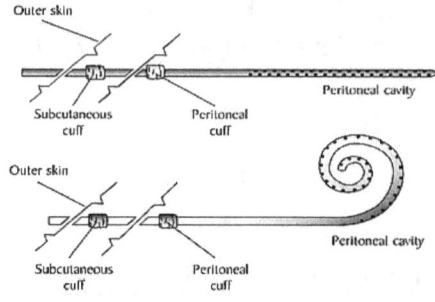

Two double-cuff Tenckhoff chronic peritoneal catheters:
standard (top), curled (bottom)

CCPD (SEE-SEE-PEE-DEE): see *continuous cycling peritoneal dialysis* under *dialysis*.

chronic (KRON-ik): refers to disorders that last a long time, often years. *Chronic kidney disease* may develop over many years and lead to *end-stage renal disease*. Chronic is the opposite of *acute*, or brief.

chronic kidney disease (CKD) (KRON-ik) (KID-nee) (dih-ZEEZ): any condition that causes reduced *kidney function* over a period of time. CKD is present when a patient's *glomerular filtration rate* remains below 60 milliliters per minute for more than 3 months or when a patient's *urine albumin-to-creatinine ratio* is over 30 milligrams (mg) of *albumin* for each gram (g) of *creatinine* (30 mg/g). CKD may develop over many years and lead to *end-stage renal disease*.

chronic kidney disease-mineral and bone disorder (CKD-MBD) (KRON-ik) (KID-nee) (dih-ZEEZ) (MIN-ur-uhl) (and) (BOHN) (dis-OR-dur): abnormal bone *hormone* levels caused by the failure of the diseased *kidneys* to maintain the proper levels of *calcium* and *phosphorus* in the blood. CKD-MBD results in weak bones, a condition known as *renal osteodystrophy*. CKD-MBD is a common problem in people with kidney disease and affects almost all patients receiving *dialysis*.

CKD (SEE-KAY-DEE): see *chronic kidney disease*.

D

dialysate (dy-AL-ih-SAYT): the part of a mixture that passes through a *semipermeable membrane*. The wastes from blood that pass into the *dialysis solution* waste. The term dialysate is sometimes used as a synonym for dialysis solution.

dialysis (dy-AL-ih-siss): the process of filtering wastes from the blood artificially. This job is normally done by the kidneys. If the kidneys fail, the blood must be filtered artificially. The two major forms of dialysis are *hemodialysis* and *peritoneal dialysis*.

hemodialysis (HEE-moh-dy-AL-ih-siss): the use of a machine to filter wastes from the blood after the *kidneys* have failed. The blood travels through tubes to a *dialyzer*, which removes wastes and extra fluid. The filtered blood then flows through another set of tubes back into the body.

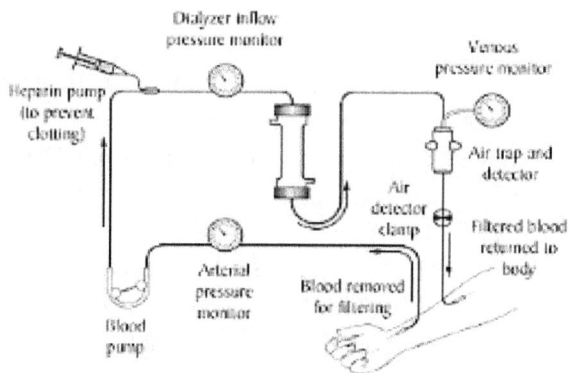

Hemodialysis

peritoneal dialysis (PAIR-ih-toh-NEE-uhl) (dy-ALih-siss): filtering the blood by using the lining of the abdominal cavity, or belly, as the filter. A cleansing liquid, called *dialysis solution*, is drained from a bag into the abdomen. Fluid and wastes flow through the lining of the abdominal cavity and remain "trapped" in the dialysis solution. The solution is then drained from the abdomen, removing the extra fluid and wastes from the body. The two main types of peritoneal dialysis are *continuous ambulatory peritoneal dialysis* and *continuous cycling peritoneal dialysis*.

continuous ambulatory peritoneal dialysis (CAPD) (kon-TIN-yoo-uhss) (AM-byoo-luh-TOR-ee) (PAIRih-toh-NEE-uhl) (dy-AL-ih-siss): a form of peritoneal dialysis that does not need a machine. With CAPD, the blood is always being filtered. The *dialysis solution* passes from a plastic bag through a *catheter* and into the abdomen. The dialysis solution stays in the abdomen with the catheter sealed. After several hours, the person using CAPD drains the solution back into a disposable bag. Then the person refills the abdomen with fresh solution through the same catheter to begin the filtering process again.

continuous cycling peritoneal dialysis (CCPD) (konTIN-yoo-uhss) (SY-kling) (PAIR-ih-toh-NEE-uhl) (dyAL-ih-siss): a form of peritoneal dialysis that uses a machine. This machine automatically fills and drains the *dialysis solution* from the abdomen. A typical CCPD schedule involves three to five *exchanges* during the night while the person sleeps. During the day, the person using CCPD performs one exchange with a *dwell time* that lasts the entire day.

dialysis solution (dy-AL-ih-siss) (suh-LOO-shuhn): a cleansing liquid used in the two major forms of *dialysis*— *hemodialysis* and *peritoneal dialysis*. Dialysis solution contains dextrose, a sugar, and other chemicals similar to those in the body. Dextrose draws wastes and extra fluid from the body into the dialysis solution. The term *dialysate* is sometimes used as a synonym for dialysis solution.

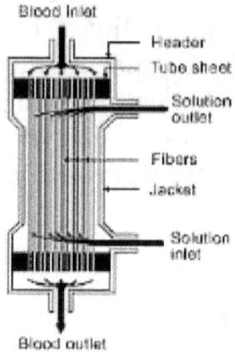

Structure of a typical hollow fiber dialyzer

dialyzer (DY-uh-LY-zur): an attachment to the *hemodialysis* machine. The dialyzer has two sections separated by a semi permeable *membrane*. One section holds *dialysis solution*. The other holds the patient's blood. See *hemodialysis* under *dialysis*.

diffusion (dih-FYOOzhuhn): the tendency of molecules packed together in a small, dense area to spread out by crossing a *semipermeable membrane* into a larger area with a lower concentration of molecules. In *dialysis*, wastes and excess *electrolytes* diffuse from the blood to the *dialysis solution*.

E

end-stage renal disease (ESRD) (END-STAYJ) (REE-nuhl) (dih-ZEEZ): total and permanent *kidney failure*. When the *kidneys* fail, the body retains fluid. Harmful wastes build up. A person with ESRD needs treatment to replace the work of the failed kidneys.

ESRD (EE-ESS-AR-DEE): see *end-stage renal disease*.

exchange (eks-CHAYNJ): in *peritoneal dialysis*, the draining of used *dialysis solution* from the abdomen, followed by refilling with a fresh bag of solution. See *peritoneal dialysis* under *dialysis*.

F

fistula (FISS-tyoo-luh): See *arteriovenous fistula*.

G

glomerulosclerosis (gloh-MAIR-yoo-loh-skluh-ROH-suhss): scarring of the *glomeruli*. It may result from *diabetes* (diabetic glomerulosclerosis) or from deposits in parts of the glomeruli (focal segmental glomerulosclerosis). The most common signs of glomerulosclerosis are *proteinuria* and *chronic kidney disease*.

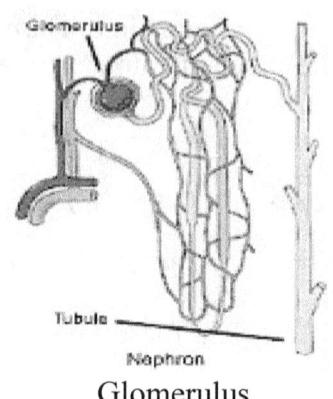

Glomerulus

glomerulus (gloh-MAIR-yoo-luhss): a tiny set of looping blood vessels in the *nephron* where blood is filtered in the *kidney*.

graft: in a *transplant*, the transplanted organ or tissue. See also *arteriovenous graft*.

H

hemodialysis (HEE-moh-dy-AL-ih-siss): See *dialysis*.

I

intravenous pyelogram (IN-truh-VEE-nuhss) (PY-el-oh-GRAM): an x ray of the *urinary tract*. A dye is injected into a *vein* in the patient's arm to make the *kidneys*, *ureters*, and *bladder* visible on the x ray and to show any blockage in the urinary tract.

K

kidney (KID-nee): one of the two bean-shaped organs that filter wastes from the blood. The kidneys are located near the middle of the back, one on each side of the spine. They create *urine*, which is delivered to the *bladder* through tubes called *ureters*.

kidney failure (KID-nee) (FAYL-yoor): loss of *kidney function*. See *end-stage renal disease*, *acute renal failure*, and *chronic kidney disease*.

kidney function (KID-nee) (FUHNK-shuhn): the amount of work done by the *kidneys*. A decline in kidney function means the kidneys are not filtering wastes and fluid from the blood as well as they should. See *glomerular filtration rate*.

Kt/V (KAY-TEE-OH-vur-VEE): a measurement of *dialysis* dose. The measurement takes into account the efficiency of the *dialyzer*, the treatment time, and the total volume of *urea* in the body. Kt/V is also used in determining the adequacy of *peritoneal dialysis*. See *urea reduction ratio*. See *peritoneal hemodialysis* under *dialysis*.

N

nephrologist (neh-FROL-uh-jist): doctor who treats people who have *kidney* problems or related conditions, such as *hypertension*.

nephrology (neh-FROL-uh-jee): a branch of medicine concerned with diseases of the *kidneys*.

P

peritoneal cavity (PAIR-ih-toh-NEE-uhl) (KAV-ih-tee): the space inside the lower abdomen but outside the internal organs.

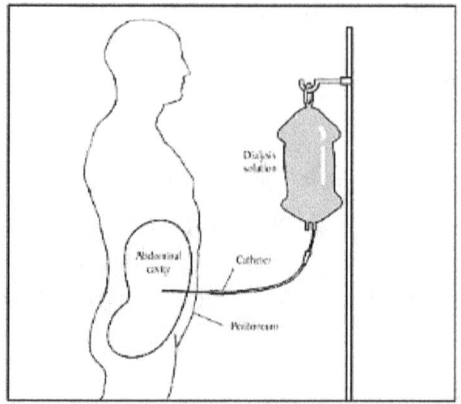

peritoneal dialysis (PAIR-ih-toh-NEE-uhl) (dy-AL-ih-siss): See *dialysis*.

peritoneum (PAIR-ih-toh-NEE-uhm): the *semipermeable membrane* lining the *peritoneal cavity*.

peritonitis (PAIR-ih-toh-NY-tiss): inflammation of the *peritoneum*, a complication of *peritoneal dialysis*. See *dialysis*.

phosphorus (FOSS-for-uhss): a mineral found in many foods, such as beans, nuts, milk, and meat.

potassium (poh-TASS-ee-uhm): a mineral and *electrolyte* found in the body and in many foods.

R

renal (REE-nuhl): of or relating to the *kidneys*. A renal disease is a disease of the kidneys. Renal failure means the kidneys are damaged.

T

thrill: a vibration or buzz that can be felt in an *arteriovenous fistula*, an indication that blood is flowing through the fistula.

U

ultrafiltration (UF) (UHL-truh-fil-TRAY-shuhn): in *dialysis*, the process by which fluid from the blood passes through a *semipermeable membrane* into a *dialysis solution*. In *peritoneal dialysis*, UF is measured as the volume of solution drained at the end of an *exchange* minus the volume of solution filled at the beginning of the exchange.

V

vascular access (VASS-kyoo-lur): a general term to describe where blood is removed from and returned to the body during *hemodialysis*. A vascular access may be an *arteriovenous fistula*, an *arteriovenous graft*, or a *catheter*. See *hemodialysis* under *dialysis*.

vein (vayn): A blood vessel that carries blood toward the heart.

venous line (VEE-nuhss) (lyn): in *hemodialysis*, tubing that carries filtered blood from the *dialyzer* back to the body. See *hemodialysis* under *dialysis*.

Glossary is provided and reprinted with permission of The National Kidney and Urologic Diseases Information Clearinghouse (NKUDIC), a service of the National Institute of Diabetes and Digestive and Kidney Diseases (NIDDK). The NIDDK is part of the National Institutes of Health of the U.S. Department of Health and Human Services.

FOR MORE INFORMATION

People on hemodialysis can learn more about how to care for an access site from their health care provider.

For information about kidney failure, or dialysis, you may contact the following resources:

National Kidney Foundation
30 East 33rd Street
New York, NY 10016–5337
Phone: 1–800–622–9010 or 212–889–2210
Fax: 212–689–9261
Internet: www.kidney.org

American Association of Kidney Patients
2701 North Rocky Point Drive, Suite 150
Tampa, FL 33607
Phone: 1–800–749–2257 or 813–636–8100
Fax: 813–636–8122
Email: info@aakp.org
Internet: www.aakp.org

The Centers for Medicare & Medicaid Services, the End-stage Renal Disease Networks, and the Institute for Healthcare Improvement launched the National Vascular Access Improvement Initiative in 2003.

PATIENT INFORMATION

It is important to keep medical information available. Some of this information changes, therefore it is advised to keep an updated list available. Current medication list is always advisable.

Patients Name: _____

Primary Care Physician: _____

Type of Dialysis Access/ Location: _____

Dialysis Clinic Location: _____

Clinic Phone Number: _____

Dialysis Days / Times: _____

Nephrologist Name: _____

Dry Weight: _____

Other medical conditions: _____

_____

List of medications as of this date: _____

Name: _____Dose/Frequency: _____

Name: _____Dose/Frequency: _____

Name: _____Dose/Frequency: _____

Name: _____Dose/Frequency: _____

ACKNOWLEDGEMENTS

Images provided by National Institute of Diabetes and Digestive and Kidney Diseases (NIDDK).

Glossary is provided and reprinted with permission of The National Kidney and Urologic Diseases Information Clearinghouse (NKUDIC), a service of the National Institute of Diabetes and Digestive and Kidney Diseases (NIDDK). The NIDDK is part of the National Institutes of Health of the U.S. Department of Health and Human Services.

"Grocery List Suggestions" for Dialysis Patients, 2004, Abbott Laboratories" and reprinted with permission of Abbott Laboratories. All registered trademarks of any products belong to their respective owners.

Some information provided by the National Kidney and Urologic Diseases Information Clearinghouse (NKUDIC).

Dr. Mark A. Kasari for editorial advice and guidance.

INDEX

nausea, 14
nephrologist
    kidney doctor, 5, 6, 7, 9,
        51, 52, 71, 72, 73, 74, 89
nephrology, 46, 90
nephron
    nephrons, 3, 4, 88
Nocturnal, 16
numb
    numbness
        numbing, 14, 73
numbing
    numb
        numbness, 9, 10, 74
    numbness
        numb, 9
pain, 9, 13, 24, 51, 74
Peritoneal, 17, 18, 19, 78
peritoneal cavity, 18, 90
peritoneum, 90
peritonitis, 90
phosphate, 2, 69
potassium, 2, 69, 77, 91
procedure center, 22, 23, 73
proteins
    protein, 3, 4

rope ladder
    rope ladder technique, 27
sodium, 2, 69
soreness
    sore, 13
swelling
    swollen, 11, 13
swollen
    swelling
        swell, 14, 75
technicians, 14
thrill, 8, 91
tubule, 3, 4
ultrasound
    angiography
        doppler, 22, 23, 24
ureters
    ureter, 1, 68, 88, 89
urethra, 1, 69
urine, 1, 3, 68, 69, 83, 89
vascular, 50, 80, 92
Vascular access
    access, 32
Vein mapping, 23
vomiting, 14